5K RUN STRONG

INTRODUCTION

Regardless of your current situation, excluding a few medically exempt people, you are capable of increasing your physical fitness more than you might realise. Much more. The obstacles standing between you and this improved fitness often seem too numerous, and therefore most people never start, or never make it past the first setback if they do. Having picked up this book though, I suspect you at least want to succeed, and that this is one of the early steps you have chosen to take. That's a good thing, because so many people choose to jump off the couch and run, without ever taking the time to think about form, distance, gradient, terrain, breathing, speed, trainers, or other things they should be doing besides just running. Whilst this book won't take care of all of that, it will definitely provide a roadmap to success, that will build a more injury resistant, stronger you when completing your 5k, that will allow you to progress to the next level, rather than ending up injured, and back where you started!

MERCH

For that extra bit of motivation, or just to show off what you're working towards, why not grab the exclusive programme t-shirt at…
www.tomhunttraining.com/shop

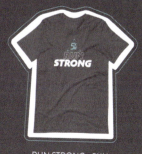

RUN STRONG - 5KM UNISEX TEE
£22.50

THE BORING BIT

Whilst the information in this book is drawn from the best research available, a myriad of specialist coaching courses with some of the best coaches in the world, and my own experience of starting running at over 112kg/247lbs body weight, to being competitive in mountain ultra-marathons, it does not constitute medical advice. You should consult with your doctor prior to commencing any physical training programme, and should not continue if you do become injured. All physical training includes an element of risk, and whilst the methods involved in this book will help to greatly reduce that risk, there is no way of completely removing it.

BEFORE YOU START

You will need a few things. Not too many, and it shouldn't be at great expense, but it pays to set yourself up for success.

A WATCH
It doesn't need to be fancy. All it needs to do is have a stopwatch function, with the ability to time laps and splits. Whilst you can use your phone, this will become inconvenient to operate at times, and a wrist worn watch is preferable. One for less than £10 should suffice.

DECENT RUNNING TRAINERS
If you haven't run for a while, chances are the casual daps you slip on for a wander around the supermarket won't be suitable. Spend a bit of time searching for some that are right for you. There are plenty of sizing guides and forums about which trainers suit which types of runner best.

MEASURED RUNNING ROUTES
Ideally where you live, and on relatively flat and even ground, you need to measure (on Google maps or similar) 100, 200, 300, 400, 800, 1000 and 1600m routes. To simplify, these can all be out and back (so the 400m run, for example, would be a point 200m away that you run to, and then back) that way you just need to add on for each additional distance.

A METHOD OF TRACKING RUNS
For the routes described above, this isn't required, however for trail runs (I know, but don't worry you will be ready) you will need an app such as Strava or similar on your phone to track your distance, time and other metrics.

A WEIGHT
This can be almost anything such as a dumbbell, kettlebell, weight plate, sandbag, or even a rucksack filled with whatever suits. The weight should suit your current ability, and you should be able to squat whilst holding it at the chest, press it overhead with one arm, and swing it from between the legs.

PROGRAMME COMPONENTS

This programme lasts for twelve weeks. It is progressive in nature, and includes not only running sessions, but bodyweight strength exercises, and some lighter loaded exercises. It assumes no start standard, other than being medically fit to participate, and targets successful completion of a 5km run without stopping at the end, rather than a specific time for that run. Other distances, such as a 10km and half marathon programme, are in the next volumes of this book, available to buy separately. The only recommendation is that you can run 400m without stopping before starting this programme.

RUNS
These will be less frequent than you might expect from a running programme. Why? Because too much, too soon is the leading cause of injury, but don't worry, the runs will be there!

STRENGTH AND CONDITIONING SESSIONS
These will be the cornerstone of the programme, and underpin its success. Sticking to these as closely as possible will set you up to reach your target.

MIXED SESSIONS
These will be new to many! A combination of strength exercises and running, that will see you progress more quickly, whilst keeping the running volume low enough not to avoid increased risk of injury.

STARTING
This bit is actually pretty easy. Most of us are excited when we start something new, and as such, motivation tends to be at a high. Whilst this is a good thing, you need to be aware that it won't last. How long it lasts will vary from person to person, we all experience times when motivation is much lower. With that in mind, creating habits now while motivation is high, will help you to have a routine to default to when things are a little tougher. Pick a time for your sessions in advance, and block them out on your calendar. Make these sessions a priority, like an important work meeting. You're prioritising your health and fitness, and the only way to stick to that, is to put it on a par with other priorities.

RUN 5K
STRONG 5M

TOM HUNT
TRAINING   05

WEEK 1

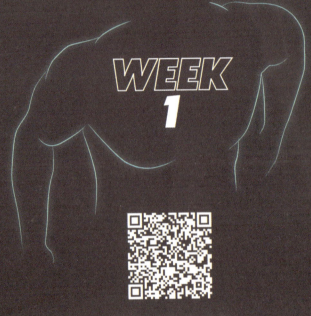

SCAN FOR VIDEO TUTORIAL

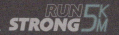

WEEK 1
DAY 1
WATCH USING QR CODE ON PAGE 06 ▶▶

WARM UP
- 5-10 MINUTES OF WALK/RUN AT A STEADY PACE.
- TOWARDS THE END, INCREASE PACE TO THE PACE YOU'RE GOING TO USE FOR THE SESSION.

THE SESSION
3-5 X 400M RUN
- TIME EACH RUN
- REST 2-3 MINUTES BETWEEN RUNS
- RECORD YOUR QUICKEST TIME AS YOUR BASELINE FOR FUTURE SESSIONS

COOL DOWN
- WALK FOR 3-5 MINUTES AFTER FINISHING THE LAST RUN
- STRETCH THE HAMSTRINGS AND CALVES AS REQUIRED

The goal here is to see how quickly you can run 400m, but with a few conditions. Firstly, follow the warm-up thoroughly, and prolong it if you don't feel ready. Secondly, use a flat route, or minimal gradient at worst. When you set off for your 400s, be a little conservative on the first one. Find your pace, and don't set expectations. Just treat your time as data, which will feed future runs. By the second and third run, you will have a handle on your ability, but even then, try to hold back 5-10% of your effort. Day 1 is not the time to push to your absolute limit! Record all times, however take particular note of your quickest run. This will become your base. If you feel cooked, or something hurts at 3 intervals, then stop. Set your ego aside, and start your cool down. If you feel okay, and you're not slowing down, then carry on to 4, or even 5 runs. Do not exceed 5, regardless of how you feel.

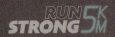

WEEK 1
DAY 2
WATCH USING QR CODE ON PAGE 06 ▶▶

WARM UP
5 X
- 5 BODYWEIGHT SQUATS
- 3 BODYWEIGHT LUNGES PER LEG
- 10 SECONDS RUNNING ON THE SPOT

THE SESSION
5 ROUNDS - NO TIME
- 10 GOBLET SQUATS
- 10 LUNGES PER LEG
- 20 SECONDS PLANK

COOL DOWN
- 30-45 SECONDS PIGEON PER LEG
- 1 MINUTE SADDLE STRETCH

Take at least 1 full day off after your first session, 2 if you need. Some soreness is normal, but outright pain is not! Day 2 targets some large movement patterns for the lower body, and a little core strength to boot. Quality and form are the keys here, not speed or weight! If you're strong enough to lift something heavy, just be aware the volume will likely still leave you sore, and may impact your training. Err on the side of caution! Move from one exercise to the next, but take around 2 minutes rest between rounds. You'll need a timer for your plank hold, and you can also use this to time the rest periods, but there's no need to time the movements themselves.

TOM HUNT TRAINING

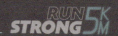

WEEK 1
DAY 3
WATCH USING QR CODE ON PAGE 06 ▶▶

WARM UP
5 X
- 10 SECONDS JOGGING ON THE SPOT
- 3 LUNGES PER LEG
- 5 TWO-FOOTED JUMPS IN PLACE

THE SESSION
RUN/WALK FOR 20 MINUTES
- RUN AT WHAT FEELS LIKE 50-60% OF YOUR BEST EFFORT, FOR AS LONG AS YOU CAN EACH TIME
- TRY TO WALK FOR NO MORE THAN 1-2 MINUTES AT A TIME
- SELECT A FLAT ROUTE WHERE POSSIBLE
- USE THE LAP TIMER TO TIME PERIODS OF RUNNING AND WALKING

COOL DOWN
- 30 SECONDS STANDING FORWARD FOLD
- 30 SECONDS PER SIDE DEEP LUNGE

Make sure you take a full day between completing day 2, and taking on day 3. On day 1, we established how quickly you can cover 400m. Today, we will establish how long you can run for, at any pace. There is a chance you can run for the whole 20 minutes. If you can, great, just don't push the pace too hard. If you can't, great, this workout is still for you! Be sure to keep a track of your total running time! Keep it to the pavements for now, and avoid hills as much as possible. Set off at what you feel is a sustainable pace, and use walks to break up periods of running. Be strict with the length of time you allow yourself to walk for though!

TOM HUNT TRAINING

1 COMPLETE
AFTER THE FIRST WEEK

How you feel right now will depend on how successful the week has been in your eyes. How you feel about your performances will largely be reflective of your expectations before starting the programme; be they conscious or unconscious. We all do it. We can't help it. We estimate our abilities and then judge our results against those estimates. The problem is, without doing something regularly, our estimates are usually way off. The more we do something, the more accurate our estimates become, as we become more aware of our own abilities. Chances are you were either shocked by the difficulty of the programme, or pleasantly surprised by how easy it was.

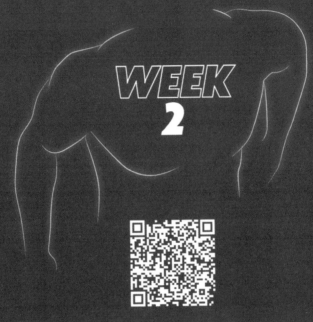

WEEK 2

SCAN FOR VIDEO TUTORIAL

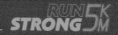

WEEK 2
DAY 1
WATCH USING QR CODE ON PAGE 12 ▶▶

WARM UP
- 5-10 MINUTES OF WALK/RUN AT A STEADY PACE.
- TOWARDS THE END, INCREASE PACE TO THE PACE YOU'RE GOING TO USE FOR THE SESSION.

THE SESSION
4-6X400M RUN
- TIME EACH RUN
- REST 2-3 MINUTES BETWEEN RUNS
- THIS SHOULD BE IDENTICAL TO LAST WEEK, HOWEVER ADD ONE RUN TO THE AMOUNT YOU DID PREVIOUSLY

COOL DOWN
- WALK FOR 3-5 MINUTES AFTER FINISHING THE LAST RUN
- STRETCH THE HAMSTRINGS AND CALVES AS REQUIRED

So now you know your pace, and what you're capable of, we're going to gradually increase your tolerance of that pace. Aim to move at the same speed as last week's best run, but add one more interval. Pretty simple, just go for it! Remember though, every day is different, so if you can't quite match your best speed, that's fine. Doing the work will still help, both physically, and mentally!

TOM HUNT TRAINING

WEEK 2
DAY 2
WATCH USING QR CODE ON PAGE 12 ▶▶

WARM UP
5 X
- 5 BODYWEIGHT SQUATS
- 3 BODYWEIGHT LUNGES PER LEG
- 10 SECONDS RUNNING ON THE SPOT
- 5 TUCK JUMPS

THE SESSION
10 MIN AMRAP*
- RUN 100M
- 10 BODYWEIGHT SQUATS
- 10 PUSH-UPS

COOL DOWN
- 30-45 SECONDS PIGEON PER LEG
- 30-45 SECONDS CRUCIFIX PER SIDE

Your first look at a mixed day. Whilst they will take differing forms, this first one is pretty simple. Set a ten minute timer, and repeat the sequence as many times as possible. The idea is to run your 100m (50m out, 50m back) then move as quickly as possible into your squats, then your push-ups, then straight back onto the run and so on. When the clock reaches ten minutes, stop, and take down your score. That might be something like 3 complete rounds plus 50m of the run. *AMRAP means As Many Rounds as Possible.

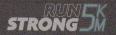

WEEK 2
DAY 3
WATCH USING QR CODE ON PAGE 12 ▶▶

WARM UP
5 X
- 10 SECONDS JOGGING ON THE SPOT
- 3 TWIST LUNGES PER LEG
- 5 SQUAT JUMPS

THE SESSION
RUN/WALK FOR 20 MINUTES
- SIMILAR TO LAST WEEK, HOWEVER THIS WEEK HEAD TO A TRAIL
- SMALL HILLS ARE OKAY, AVOID BIG ONES
- TARGET RUNNING FOR 1 MINUTE MORE THAN LAST WEEK

COOL DOWN
- 30 SECONDS STANDING FORWARD FOLD
- 30 SECONDS PER SIDE DEEP LUNGE

Select somewhere visually attractive, away from urban areas and mixed terrain if possible. If that's not possible, do the best you can. Why? Running in nice places is always so much more enjoyable, and distracts from the discomfort caused by the activity. Why do we run on trails? The changing surface helps to build stability, strength and resilience in our ankles and legs. This is all part of reducing injury risk. Additionally, the natural surface is a lot more forgiving than concrete, and this helps too! Whilst you will probably encounter a couple of little hills, avoid anything too big. Use hills as an opportunity to walk, remembering that the goal is to run for just slightly more of that 20 minute window than you did last week.

2 COMPLETE
TWO WEEKS IN

So be honest, this probably isn't as bad as you thought, is it? Depending on how you tend to estimate tasks, you're probably pleasantly surprised by how well you're adapting. If not, take an honest look at your food and recovery. It's beyond the scope of this book to delve into those two particularly important subjects, however suffice it to say that you need to be eating well enough (quality) and enough (quantity) to support your new routine. Sleeping 7.5-9 hours per night is also a near universal recommendation, and one you should follow as well as you can to maximise recovery, and minimise your chances of sustaining an injury, or becoming run down and ill. You will notice, by looking ahead, that things do begin to pick up pace a little. Don't worry though, you are already a different person than you were two weeks back, and can already handle more. Remember, you have earned the right to do more, by getting this far!

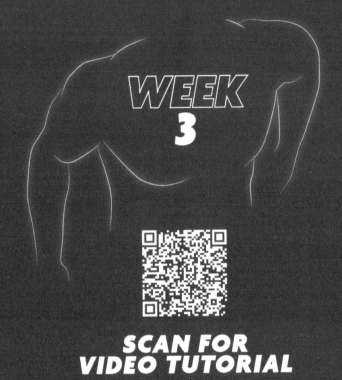

WEEK 3

SCAN FOR VIDEO TUTORIAL

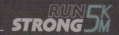

WEEK 3
DAY 1
WATCH USING QR CODE ON PAGE 18 ▶▶

WARM UP
- 5-10 MINUTES OF WALK/RUN AT A STEADY PACE.
- TOWARDS THE END, INCREASE PACE TO THE PACE YOU'RE GOING TO USE FOR THE SESSION AND INCORPORATE HIGH KNEES AND HEEL FLICKS

THE SESSION
4-6 X 400M + 20 WALKING LUNGES
- TIME EACH RUN
- REST 2-3 MINUTES BETWEEN RUNS
- COMPLETE THE SAME NUMBER OF RUNS AS LAST WEEK
- IMMEDIATELY AFTER FINISHING EACH RUN, MOVE STRAIGHT INTO THE WALKING LUNGES. THERE SHOULD BE NO GAP BETWEEN RUNS AND LUNGES
- THE LUNGES SHOULD BE PERFORMED AT A MODERATE PACE, WHILST BREATHING IS RECOVERED
- THE LUNGES ARE INCLUDED WITHIN THE REST TIME, WHICH STARTS AS SOON AS THE RUN IS FINISHED

COOL DOWN
- WALK FOR 3-5 MINUTES AFTER FINISHING THE LAST RUN
- STRETCH THE HAMSTRINGS AND CALVES AS REQUIRED

Whilst this is a running focused session, the increase this week doesn't come in volume, speed or intensity, but by adding a challenge into the recovery period. Learning to recover without coming to a complete stop is a valuable skill, and ultimately helps us recover more effectively. Time per run should remain constant, and should be the same as previous weeks, and the rest period should remain constant too. Don't rush the lunges, rather focus on trying to return the breathing to normal whilst performing them at a controlled pace. Once the lunges are complete, continue the remainder of the rest period standing tall, focusing on breathing.

WEEK 3
DAY 2
WATCH USING QR CODE ON PAGE 18 ▶▶

WARM UP
5 X
- 3 WALKOUTS
- 3 BURPEES
- 5 ARM CIRCLES EACH DIRECTION

THE SESSION
7 ROUNDS FOR TIME*
- RUN 200M
- 8 BURPEES
- 16 THRUSTERS

COOL DOWN
- 30-45 SECONDS PIGEON PER LEG
- 30-45 SECONDS SEATED SHOULDER STRETCH

Another mixed day, and one where we really begin to target intensity. The aim is to get through the prescribed work, whilst maintaining good form, as quickly as possible. Much like the 5km run you're aiming for at the end of this programme, the incentive is the more quickly you move, the quicker it's done! Be sure to use the video to correctly adapt the workout to your ability level to ensure you avoid injury, but maintain the desired effect by completing the movements properly.
*Rounds for Time means complete the work written the stated number of times, as quickly as possible.

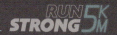

WEEK 3
DAY 3
WATCH USING QR CODE ON PAGE 18 ▶▶

WARM UP
5 X
- 50M JOG
- 10 BODYWEIGHT SQUATS
- 10 OSTRICH STEPS

THE SESSION
3-4 X RUN 800M
- RATHER THAN OUT AND BACK AT HOME, HEAD TO THE TRAIL AGAIN
- THESE 800M RUNS DO NOT NEED TO BE THE SAME EACH TIME
- AFTER EACH 800M RUN, WALK FOR 3-4 MINUTES AT A STEADY PACE
- DURING THE RUNS, LEAVE A LITTLE IN THE TANK, THEY SHOULD NOT BE BEST EFFORT, BUT AROUND 70-80%.
- AFTER THE FINAL RUN, PERFORM 3 PLANK HOLDS, EACH FOR AS LONG AS POSSIBLE, WITH A 2 MINUTE BREAK BETWEEN.
- REST 2 MINUTES AFTER THE FINAL RUN, BEFORE THE FIRST PLANK HOLD

COOL DOWN
- 30 SECONDS STANDING FORWARD FOLD
- 30 SECONDS COSSACK PER SIDE

Get back to that trail, and get ready to get dirty! More ankle and calf strengthening, along with more time out in the countryside. A slight change with this session. We are performing intervals, but with the aim of completing longer runs, rather than setting speed records. Pace doesn't matter here, as it's likely each 800m run will be different, so base this more off your own perception of effort. Run at 70-80% until 800m is complete, then walk at a steady pace whilst recovering the breathing. The goal is to avoid coming to a standstill. Be sure to walk for at least a minute or two after the last run, before resting and beginning the plank holds.

3 COMPLETE

THIS MIGHT SEEM CRAZY BUT...

...you're already a quarter of the way through this programme! If you're anything like me when I first found fitness, three weeks is probably the longest you have stuck with a positive habit change? If that's you too, well done! If it's not, still well done. Regardless, this is three weeks of positive change, commitment, and moving towards a goal that you have chosen. Additionally, you're at that mythical 21 day point where habits start to become ingrained. Take a moment to look back over your training to date, and don't be afraid to pat yourself on the back! That said, in the words of Max Lerner, "Satisfaction is the death of desire.". In other words, be happy with what you have done so far, but don't let that be enough. Week 4 is just around the corner, and you now have all the tools you need to take it on, and succeed.

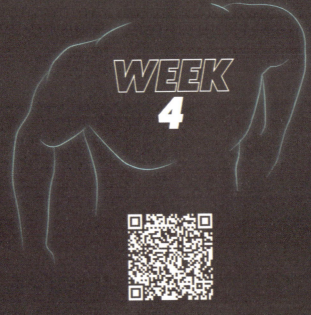

WEEK 4

SCAN FOR VIDEO TUTORIAL

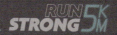

WEEK 4
DAY 1
WATCH USING QR CODE ON PAGE 24 ▶▶

WARM UP
- 5-10 MINUTES OF WALK/RUN AT A STEADY PACE.
- TOWARDS THE END, INCREASE PACE TO THE PACE YOU'RE GOING TO USE FOR THE SESSION AND INCORPORATE HIGH KNEES AND HEEL FLICKS

THE SESSION
3-4 X 600M + 20 WALKING LUNGES
- TIME EACH RUN
- REST 2-3 MINUTES BETWEEN RUNS
- KEEP THE REST THE SAME AS PREVIOUS WEEKS

COOL DOWN
- WALK FOR 3-5 MINUTES AFTER FINISHING THE LAST RUN
- STRETCH THE HAMSTRINGS AND CALVES AS REQUIRED

This week, distance goes up per interval, but total distance remains the same. Rest remains the same, and all being well, speed remains similar too. Keep the lunges in to help the body learn to recover more efficiently. It would be ideal if the 600m route you used incorporated the 400m route from previous weeks, so we have a constant surface to maintain pace over.

WEEK 4
DAY 2
WATCH USING QR CODE ON PAGE 24 ▶▶

WARM UP
5 X
- 3 WALKOUTS
- 10 ALTERNATING ARM CIRCLES
- 10 EMPTY PRESS

THE SESSION
4 X
- 8 STRICT PRESS PER ARM
- 10 GOOD MORNINGS
- 12 GOBLET SQUATS
- 14 SIT-UPS

FOR TIME
- 8 STRICT PRESS PER ARM
- 10 GOOD MORNINGS
- 12 GOBLET SQUATS
- 14 SIT-UPS

COOL DOWN
- 1 MINUTE SAMSON STRETCH
- 1 MINUTE UPDOG
- 1 MIN SADDLE

In a bit of a twist, this week sees some strength work without a time component, into a timed workout. It is vital you conduct a mini warm-up after the strength work, before the timed workout! Focus on form and strength building for the first part, using the weight you have available to the best of your ability. Ensure you support the lumbar fully during sit-ups as shown in the video! Whilst the workout is relatively short, you must ensure to adapt it appropriately in order to get maximum benefit. This should be a fast pace, and stay fast throughout. The aim is to avoid hitting a wall part way through! *For Time simply means complete the work written as quickly as possible.

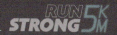

WEEK 4
DAY 3
WATCH USING QR CODE ON PAGE 24 ▶▶

WARM UP
5 X
- 50M JOG
- 10 WALKING LUNGES
- 10 SECONDS HIGH KNEES

THE SESSION
RUN 2KM, WALK 2KM
- ON THE TRAIL, RUN AT A SUSTAINABLE PACE FOR 2KM
- AVOID STOPPING AT ALL COSTS
- AVOID HILLS TO HELP WITH THIS
- AS SOON AS YOU HIT 2KM, CONTINUE TO WALK FOR 2KM WITH NO BREAK
- WALK AT A CHALLENGING PACE, AND FEEL FREE TO INCLUDE SOME HILLS

COOL DOWN
- 45 SECONDS STANDING FORWARD FOLD
- 45 SECONDS DEEP LUNGE

More time on the trail, and your longest non-stop run to date (potentially, depending on your twenty minute run-walk results). Do everything you can to set yourself up for success. Plan a flat route on good, open trails. Set off at a pace you're confident can last, and only increase the pace once you know you can complete the 2km. As soon as your tracking app or watch indicates you have completed 2km, move straight into a challenging pace walk. As fast as this might be, really work to reduce the breathing rate whilst walking. Depending on your location, you can turn around and walk back to the start, or continue on a different route to loop back. If the route is different, include a hill or to to challenge your recovery even more.

TOM HUNT TRAINING

4 COMPLETE
BUT WHY TRAILS?

When people see the miles I run, or how often I run, they find it a little odd that I then tell them I don't like running. In comparison to most 'runners' I really don't run very often, or very fast, however to someone who doesn't run, it may seem that I do. Most can wrap their heads around this concept, but still fail to see why I run at all if I don't enjoy it. The truth is relatively simple, firstly I enjoy being fit and the things that being fit allows me to do. Running is a staple of any fitness programme. Secondly, and probably more importantly, running allows me access to experiences that I can't get in any other way. At any time, with nothing more than a reasonable level of hydration, and a pair of trainers and shorts, I can step out of the front door of my house, work or car, and be running. I can access spots only open to those on foot and, because it is quicker than walking, cover far more distance, or the same distance much more quickly, than if I were to walk. I've run coastal paths, mountains, woodland trails, public footpaths and untrodden and buried trails. I dislike the act of running. I don't enjoy running 400 or 800m repeats on the pavement. However, I do enjoy the feeling it gives me, and I particularly enjoy the trails and remote views and wilderness that the fitness generated gives me access to. That's why when I wrote this programme, I was extremely keen to encourage participants to get out to the trails, and discover just a snippet of what's on offer with just a small increase in fitness. Add in the injury reducing properties of trail running, and the question I would ask is, why not trails?

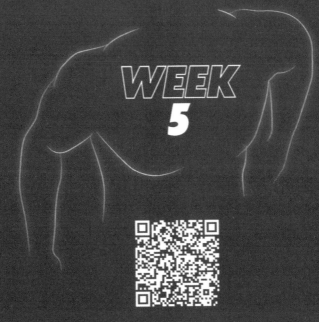

WEEK 5

SCAN FOR VIDEO TUTORIAL

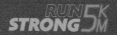

WEEK 5
DAY 1
WATCH USING QR CODE ON PAGE 30 ▸▸

WARM UP
- 5-10 MINUTES OF WALK/RUN AT A STEADY PACE.
- TOWARDS THE END, INCREASE PACE TO THE PACE YOU'RE GOING TO USE FOR THE SESSION AND INCORPORATE HIGH KNEES AND HEEL FLICKS

THE SESSION
4-5 X 600M + 20 WALKING LUNGES
- TIME EACH RUN
- REST 2-3 MINUTES BETWEEN RUNS
- KEEP THE REST THE SAME AS PREVIOUS WEEKS
- THE NUMBER OF REPS HAS INCREASED BY ONE, BUT TRY TO KEEP THE SAME PACE AS LAST WEEK, AND THE 400M RUNS FROM PREVIOUS WEEKS

COOL DOWN
- WALK FOR 3-5 MINUTES AFTER FINISHING THE LAST RUN
- STRETCH THE HAMSTRINGS AND CALVES AS REQUIRED

This week, we just add one more run. No change to pace, rest or anything else. Be sure to hold yourself accountable to the pace, and that extra rep!

TOM HUNT TRAINING

WEEK 5
DAY 2
WATCH USING QR CODE ON PAGE 30 ▶▶

WARM UP
5 X
- 20 HIGH KNEES
- 10 BODYWEIGHT SQUATS
- 20 ALTERNATING TOE TAPS

THE SESSION
4 X
- 10 STRICT PRESS PER ARM
- 12 GOOD MORNINGS
- 14 GOBLET SQUATS
- 16 SIT-UPS

5 ROUNDS FOR TIME
- 5 BURPEES
- 10 GOBLET SQUATS
- 15 SIT-UPS
- STAIR CLIMB

COOL DOWN
- 1 MINUTE GROIN STRETCH
- 30 SECONDS DEEP LUNGE
- 30 SECONDS CRUCIFIX

Continuing on from last week, you again start with some strength work. Here the aim is to maintain the same standard as last week, but add 2 reps to each movement. Keep the weight the same if at all possible. For the workout, the pace and intensity should be high. If you don't have stairs available, you can perform 10 tuck jumps instead. Full adaptations and instructions are available in the video.

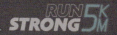

WEEK 5
DAY 3
WATCH USING QR CODE ON PAGE 30 ▶▶

WARM UP
5 X
- 50M JOG
- 10 WALKING LUNGES
- 10 SECONDS HIGH KNEES
- THEN JOG TO START (500M-1KM)

THE SESSION
4-6 X 150M HILL REPS
- FIND A NEARBY HILL WITH AN ACHIEVABLE GRADIENT
- FROM THE BOTTOM, RUN HARD UP, THEN TURN AROUND AND JOG BACK DOWN
- AT THE BOTTOM, IMMEDIATELY BEGIN THE NEXT RUN
- AFTER THE FINAL RUN, JOG/WALK BACK TO STRETCH
- TIME EACH REP, BUT DON'T WORRY ABOUT THE JOGS BACK DOWN

COOL DOWN
- 45 SECONDS STANDING CALF STRETCH
- 45 SECONDS DEEP LUNGE

This week sees the introduction of hill reps for the first time. Hill reps are particularly challenging, because the amount gravity assists us decreases, and the demand on our legs, especially quadriceps and calves, increases. This effect is greater, the steeper the hill. Select somewhere 500m-1km from your house (or travel to somewhere appropriate) and, after the short warm-up, jog to the start to continue your warm-up. Pace or measure out 150m. This doesn't need to be exact, but does need to be repeatable in coming weeks. Run as hard as you can from bottom to top, then jog as slowly as you like back to the start. Time each run with a watch. If you slow by more than 5 seconds, stop at 4 reps, but if you maintain speed, continue to 5 or 6. The idea is not to walk at all, although your recovery down the hill can be as slow a jog as you like. After the last run, jog back the same distance as your warm-up, to the start to begin your cooldown.

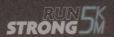

WEEK 5
DAY 4
WATCH USING QR CODE ON PAGE 30 ▶▶

WARM UP
- 5-10 MINUTES OF WALK/RUN AT A STEADY PACE.
- TOWARDS THE END, INCREASE PACE TO THE PACE YOU'RE GOING TO USE FOR THE SESSION AND INCORPORATE TOE SWEEPS AND HIGH KNEES

THE SESSION
RUN 3-4KM
- THIS IS A RECOVERY RUN, AND SHOULD BE PERFORMED AT 50-60% EFFORT
- SOME WALKING IS OKAY, BUT KEEP IT TO A MINIMUM
- BE ABLE TO TALK IN FULL SENTENCES THROUGHOUT

COOL DOWN
- 1 MINUTE DEEP BAND/STRAP HAMSTRING STRETCH
- 1 MINUTE SADDLE

Wait. What? Yes, a fourth day. You have earned it. You see, you're already fitter, more efficient at recovering, and healthier than when you started. The problem is, if we keep doing the same amount, that progress won't last. Adding another session is just one more way of ensuring progress. So here goes! Nice and steady for this. Don't worry if you need a walk, but do be strict with yourself, and get back to running as soon as you're able. If 3km sounds like a lot, stick to that, but if you're able, shoot for that 4km mark. Whatever you do, DO NOT push the pace today. Take it easy, then enjoy a deep stretch afterwards.

TOM HUNT TRAINING

5 COMPLETE

BUT WHY RESISTANCE TRAINING?

Running is fantastic. It is great for our heart and lungs, great for the muscular endurance of our lower bodies, and a great tool for getting us outside. It is probably our oldest form of exercise, albeit our ancient ancestors wouldn't have seen it as exercise. That all sounds great, but there are some drawbacks. Firstly, running has quite a high injury rate. This high rate is usually associated with minor injuries, and usually stems from either doing too much too soon, running with poor form, or by not having the required muscle and tendon strength to support the movement. Strength training, notably resistance training, helps with all of this except for maybe running form. Resistance training performed properly takes our joints through a full range of motion, whereas running is only a partial range of motion exercise. Additionally, it builds muscle and tendon strength and increases bone density, which helps in turn with better posture, movement, and resistance to injury. Additionally, if you are unlucky enough to still get injured, your recovery time will be shorter if you are stronger and better conditioned. Also, as our need to train more often becomes apparent, strength training is much lower impact than running, which gives our body a valuable session, without the volume of impact we are subjected to in a longer running session. As with my question about why not trails, I say again here: why not resistance training?

WEEK 6

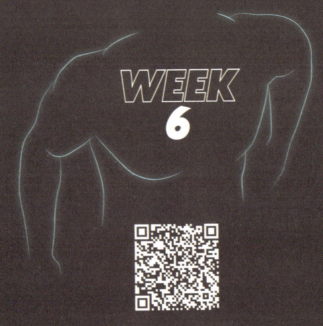

SCAN FOR VIDEO TUTORIAL

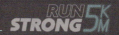

WEEK 6
DAY 1
WATCH USING QR CODE ON PAGE 36 ▶▶

WARM UP
- 5-10 MINUTES OF WALK/RUN AT A STEADY PACE.
- TOWARDS THE END, INCREASE PACE TO THE PACE YOU'RE GOING TO USE FOR THE SESSION AND INCORPORATE SHORT SPRINTS AND TURNS

THE SESSION
4-5X600M+20 WALKING LUNGES
- TIME EACH RUN
- REST 1-2 MINUTES BETWEEN RUNS
- COMPLETE THE SAME NUMBER OF RUNS AS LAST WEEK
- REDUCE THE REST BY 1 MINUTE FROM PREVIOUS WEEKS
- AIM TO MAINTAIN PACE, EVEN WITH THE REDUCTION IN REST
- MAINTAINING PACE FROM PREVIOUS WEEKS MAY NOT BE POSSIBLE, BUT KEEP PACE THROUGHOUT

COOL DOWN
- WALK FOR 3-5 MINUTES AFTER FINISHING THE LAST RUN
- STRETCH THE HAMSTRINGS AND CALVES AS REQUIRED

You've started to build a solid tolerance for volume, now we look at recovering more efficiently. Knocking a full minute off your rest time is a big ask, but you can do it. If your pace drops a little, that's fine for now. Do hold yourself to the same pace each round though, and don't let your head defeat you. This one is in the mind!

WEEK 6
DAY 2
WATCH USING QR CODE ON PAGE 36 ▶▶

WARM UP
5 X
- 3 WALKOUT TO UPDOG
- 3 BURPEES
- 3 CRUCIFIX ROLLS PER SIDE

THE SESSION
4 X
- 10 FLOOR PRESS
- 10 UPRIGHT ROWS
- 10 PUSH PRESS
- 10 BENT OVER ROWS

12 MIN EMOM*
- 2 STAIR CLIMBS
- 5 BURPEES
- 5 BODYWEIGHT SQUATS

COOL DOWN
- 1 MINUTE PIGEON STRETCH
- 1 MINUTE RAISED CALF STRETCH

A shift in exercises this week, but still aimed at building strength. Remember, to get the most out of these movements, you need to move well, so be sure to watch the video before getting started. EMOMs are a great way to earn your rest; the more quickly you complete the work each minute, the more rest you get before starting again the next minute. Set a watch, and work through your stair climbs, burpees and squats as quickly as possible, without losing form, and then rest until the minute is up. At the start of the next minute, repeat this process. Complete twelve rounds of this in total. *EMOM means Every Minute On the Minute complete the work as quickly as possible, then rest until the start of the next minute.

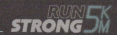

WEEK 6
DAY 3
WATCH USING QR CODE ON PAGE 36 ▶▶

WARM UP
5 X
- 20M HIGH KNEES
- 20M HEEL FLICKS
- 20M TOE SWEEPS
- THEN BUILD RUNNING PACE

THE SESSION
RUN: 1200M, 1000M, 800M, 600M
- RUN THE 1200M AT ALMOST YOUR BEST PACE, THINK 90% EFFORT OR ABOVE
- DIVIDE YOUR TIME BY 6 (TO GIVE YOU YOUR PACE PER 200M)
- REST THE SAME TIME AS THE PREVIOUS RUN, BEFORE THE NEXT RUN
- THE 1000, 800 AND 600M RUNS SHOULD BE AT THE SAME, OR FASTER, PACE PER 200M AS THE 1200M

COOL DOWN
- 1 MINUTE STANDING FORWARD FOLD
- 1 MINUTE BANDED PANCAKE
- 30 SECONDS SPRINT CALF STRETCH

Decreasing intervals are great at allowing us to squeeze as much effort and speed out of a session as possible. The first run sets the standard, because if you can hold it for 1200m, you know you can hold it for less than that! With a slightly more generous rest period - the same length of time as the previous run took - we can push the pace a bit this week. Think 90% or above for that first run. 1200m is approximately ¾ mile, and gives you a nice benchmark time for the future.

TOM HUNT TRAINING

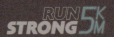

WEEK 6
DAY 4
WATCH USING QR CODE ON PAGE 36 ▶▶

WARM UP
- 5-10 MINUTES OF WALK/RUN AT A STEADY PACE.
- TOWARDS THE END, INCREASE PACE TO THE PACE YOU'RE GOING TO USE FOR THE SESSION AND INCORPORATE TOE SWEEPS AND HIGH KNEES

THE SESSION
RUN 3/4 KM
- THIS IS A RECOVERY RUN, AND SHOULD BE PERFORMED AT 50-60% EFFORT
- SOME WALKING IS OKAY, BUT KEEP IT TO A MINIMUM
- THIS SHOULD BE THE SAME DISTANCE AND PACE AS LAST WEEK

COOL DOWN
- 1 MINUTE DEEP BAND/STRAP HAMSTRING STRETCH
- 1 MINUTE SADDLE

With an exact repeat of last week, it is important to remember that there is no desire to run more quickly, or for longer this week. This run serves as recovery, and helps to flush blood through sore muscles. Avoid the temptation to try and improve. If it helps, turn your tracker off and just use a simple stopwatch on a pre-measured route.

TOM HUNT TRAINING

6 COMPLETE

PHYSICAL VERSUS MENTAL

One of my goals as a coach is to make people realise that those who do extraordinary things, achieve unbelievable physical feats and break seemingly impossible barriers, are just like you and I. The only difference is that for a considerable period of time, they have committed themselves to a routine, and achieving small daily tasks, that have combined to put them in a position to take on the world. Former John O'Groats to Lands End world record holder, Mimi Anderson, started as a housewife on a treadmill looking to get into slightly better shape. Christopher McDougall, author of "Born to Run", was once overweight and couldn't run more than a few hundred metres without excruciating pain. Some of McDougall's characters in "Natural Born Heroes" repeatedly covered 50+ miles through the mountains of Crete in World War 2, whilst carrying supplies. My take on it is pretty simple; you have two mental challenges. Firstly you have to decide you want to improve. Secondly, you have to decide to do the things that make that improvement happen. It always sounds so much more simple than it is in practice, but often that's because we allow ourselves to imagine obstacles that aren't really there, or magnify small ones in our mind until they become insurmountable. That tiny sore spot on your big toe as you run will definitely require an amputation. Your breathlessness is most definitely a sign that you are only seconds from death. The smattering of snow on the ground means you can't possibly leave the house and return alive. The point is, mental strength allows us to begin, and by beginning we create physical change. This is why, for me, mental strength underpins physical progress.

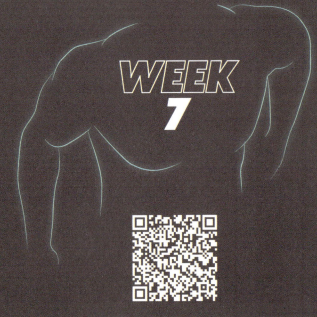

WEEK 7

SCAN FOR VIDEO TUTORIAL

WEEK 7
DAY 1
WATCH USING QR CODE BELOW ▶▶

THE SESSION
ONLINE STRETCH FLOW
- LOG INTO THE WATCH LINK USING THE QR CODE BELOW TO FOLLOW ALONG.

SCAN FOR VIDEO TUTORIAL

We're taking the foot off the gas a little this week. A chance to reset, and recover more. Eat well, get extra sleep and focus on a slower pace of life and movement. After 6 weeks in a new programme, the body will be sore, and the nervous system will be adapting at a rapid rate. We're going to take a week to let them catch up. Follow the flows, and make the most of some down time.

WEEK 7
DAY 2
WATCH USING QR CODE ON PAGE 42 ▶▶

WARM UP
- 3-4 MINUTES WALK INTO JOG
- 2 MINUTES OF TOE SWEEPS, HIGH KNEES AND HIP OPENERS

THE SESSION
RUN FOR 25 MINUTES
- 25 MINUTES AT AN EVEN PACE
- AROUND 60-70% EFFORT
- AVOID TOO MANY, OR PARTICULARLY STEEP HILLS
- USE A TRAIL IF POSSIBLE

COOL DOWN
- 1 MINUTE SEATED HAMSTRING STRETCH
- 1 MINUTE RAISED CALF STRETCH

If you're able to get to the trail, great, if not the pavements will still be fine. Keep the pace low, and focus on moving. If 25 minutes seems a little long, bring it down to 20 minutes, and use walking breaks as required. Take this opportunity to unplug from metrics and data, and focus on breathing and enjoying your surroundings.

WEEK 7
DAY 3
WATCH USING QR CODE BELOW ▶▶

THE SESSION
ONLINE STRETCH FLOW
- LOG INTO THE WATCH LINK USING THE QR CODE BELOW TO FOLLOW ALONG.

SCAN FOR VIDEO TUTORIAL

WEEK 7
DAY 4
WATCH USING QR CODE ON PAGE 42 ▶▶

WARM UP
- 3-4 MINUTES WALK INTO JOG
- 2 MINUTES OF TOE SWEEPS, HIGH KNEES AND HIP OPENERS

THE SESSION
RUN FOR 25 MINUTES
- 25 MINUTES AT AN EVEN PACE
- AROUND 60-70% EFFORT
- AVOID TOO MANY, OR PARTICULARLY STEEP HILLS
- USE A TRAIL IF POSSIBLE

COOL DOWN
- 1 MINUTE STANDING FORWARD FOLD
- 1 MIN SADDLE

If you're able to get to the trail, great, if not the pavements will still be fine. Keep the pace low, and focus on moving. If 25 minutes seems a little long, bring it down to 20 minutes, and use walking breaks as required. Take this opportunity to unplug from metrics and data, and focus on breathing and enjoying your surroundings.

7 COMPLETE

THIS WEEK PROBABLY FELT WEIRD

6 weeks is a long time to be in a routine for. Routines are hard to implement, but easy to neglect and lose. For that reason, even though the intensity has stepped right back, the routine remains. Habits are one of the most powerful functions our brain performs, to the point we simply couldn't imagine life without them. How much thought do you put into brushing your teeth, or pulling on clean underwear each day? What about starting your car engine or the act of sitting down? These are small tasks repeated so often, that the brain goes into autopilot and performs them with minimal mental effort. Hacking into these loops is powerful, because in the contemplation of an upcoming task, lies the opportunity to find an excuse not to do it. By removing the conscious thought required to go and run, or to go and workout, by habituating it, we remove that opportunity. Sticking with your routine this week has helped to reinforce those habit loops, whilst providing some much needed recovery.

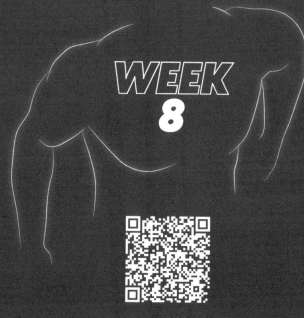

WEEK 8

SCAN FOR VIDEO TUTORIAL

WEEK 8
DAY 1
WATCH USING QR CODE ON PAGE 48 ▶▶

WARM UP
- 5-10 MINUTES OF WALK/RUN AT A STEADY PACE.
- TOWARDS THE END, INCREASE PACE TO THE PACE YOU'RE GOING TO USE FOR THE SESSION AND INCORPORATE SHORT SPRINTS AND TURNS

THE SESSION
2-3 X 1000M + 30 WALKING LUNGES
- TIME EACH RUN
- REST 2-3 MINUTES BETWEEN RUNS
- REST INCREASES AGAIN, BUT SO DOES DISTANCE COMPARED TO PREVIOUS WEEKS
- NOTE THE INCREASE IN LUNGES, WHICH REMAIN INCLUDED IN THE REST TIME
- AIM TO MAINTAIN PACE, ALTHOUGH A SMALL DROP OFF IS PERFECTLY OKAY

COOL DOWN
- WALK FOR 3-5 MINUTES AFTER FINISHING THE LAST RUN
- STRETCH THE HAMSTRINGS AND CALVES AS REQUIRED

More distance per rep, more lunges, but also a little more rest again. The volume is starting to accumulate, but not too much. This is within your new found abilities, so you have earned the right to take on a session like this. Aim for near identical times on each run, and remember to watch the video for tips on how to spend your rest periods.

WEEK 8
DAY 2
WATCH USING QR CODE ON PAGE 48 ▶▶

WARM UP
5 X
- 10 CHEST OPENERS
- 10 EMPTY PRESS
- 10 WINDMILLS

THE SESSION
4 X
- 12 FLOOR PRESS
- 12 UPRIGHT ROWS
- 12 PUSH PRESS
- 12 BENT OVER ROWS

4 X
- 12 BURPEES
- 24 WALKING LUNGES
- 36 MOUNTAIN CLIMBERS
- 48 POGO HOPS

COOL DOWN
- 1 MINUTE STANDING CALF STRETCH
- 1 MINUTE SEATED SHOULDER STRETCH

A few more reps on exercises you have visited before, then a gnarly workout. This is designed to get the heart pumping and the breath a little erratic. Go with it, and hold on to your form despite the urge to break posture and breathe hard. For full modification tips, be sure to watch the video. Move hard, and enjoy a shorter, sprint style workout!

WEEK 8
DAY 3
WATCH USING QR CODE ON PAGE 48 ▶▶

WARM UP
3 X
- RUN 200M
- 30M HIGH KNEES
- 30M HEEL FLICKS
- 30M RUN HARD

THE SESSION
RUN 3.5KM
- RUN AT 80-90% EFFORT - LEAVE A LITTLE IN THE TANK
- AVOID HILLS AND ROAD CROSSINGS
- STICK TO EVEN PAVEMENT SURFACE
- TRY TO MAINTAIN PACE THROUGHOUT, AND AVOID THE TEMPTATION TO FINISH HARD

COOL DOWN
- 1 MINUTE BAND OR STRAP HAMSTRING STRETCH
- 1 MINUTE SADDLE
- 30 SECONDS SPRINT CALF STRETCH

We're pretty much two thirds done, and that means a time trial! We're not quite going flat out though. At this stage, you should have a reasonable understanding of your pace, and what you can sustain. This should be tough, but you should be able to run around another 500-100m at the same pace if you had to. Again, even pacing is the aim, but be aware that will feel easier at the start than the end. Log your time carefully. At 70% of the distance you're training for, this will serve as a great comparison in a few weeks! Stick to pavement, avoid road crossings, and be thorough with your warm up!

WEEK 8
DAY 4
WATCH USING QR CODE ON PAGE 48 ▶▶

WARM UP
- 5-10 MINUTES OF WALK/RUN AT A STEADY PACE.
- TOWARDS THE END, INCREASE PACE TO THE PACE YOU'RE GOING TO USE FOR THE SESSION AND INCORPORATE TOE SWEEPS AND HIGH KNEES

THE SESSION
RUN FOR 30 MINUTES
- THIS IS A RECOVERY RUN, AND SHOULD BE PERFORMED AT 50-60% EFFORT
- SOME WALKING IS OKAY, BUT KEEP IT TO A MINIMUM
- THIS SHOULD BE ON THE TRAIL IF POSSIBLE

COOL DOWN
- 1 MINUTE DEEP BAND/STRAP HAMSTRING STRETCH
- 1 MINUTE COSSACK

Targeting time instead of distance is great for pacing. It makes it easier to project out, and in theory it is easier to run for time, when we aren't trying to do our best. A couple of hills are fine, but keep that effort level low to moderate, think being able to speak in sentences throughout.

8 COMPLETE
NORMALITY RESUMES

You probably found yourself grateful for the return of some intensity this week, and also probably surprised yourself with how much energy you had. This has served a couple of purposes; it allowed you to physically recover, but it also taught you that a week away from pushing yourself 3-4 times per week, doesn't mean you lose all of the fitness you worked so hard for. Take the recovery flow you used this week, and add it in as a bonus session in the coming weeks, if your body starts to feel overly tired or tight.

WEEK 9

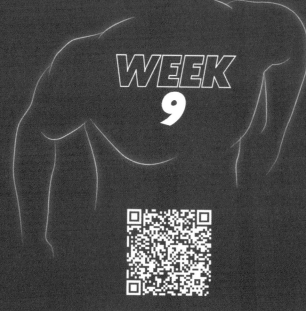

SCAN FOR
VIDEO TUTORIAL

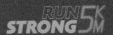

WEEK 9
DAY 1
WATCH USING QR CODE ON PAGE 54 ▶▶

WARM UP
- 5-10 MINUTES OF WALK/RUN AT A STEADY PACE.
- TOWARDS THE END, INCREASE PACE TO THE PACE YOU'RE GOING TO USE FOR THE SESSION AND INCORPORATE SHORT SPRINTS AND TURNS

THE SESSION
RUN: 1600M, 1200M, 800M, 400M
- TIME EACH RUN
- REST THE SAME TIME AS THE PREVIOUS RUN BEFORE RUNNING AGAIN
- RUN THE FIRST 1600M (1 MILE) AT ALMOST BEST EFFORT TO ESTABLISH A TIME (LOG THIS AS 1 MILE RECORD)
- DIVIDE THE 1600M TIME BY 4 TO GET YOU PACE PER 400M
- FOR THE REMAINDER OF THE RUNS, AIM TO MATCH OR BEAT THE 400M PACE OF THE FIRST RUN

COOL DOWN
- WALK FOR 3-5 MINUTES AFTER FINISHING THE LAST RUN
- STRETCH THE HAMSTRINGS AND CALVES AS REQUIRED

Decreasing distance again, meaning we can hold that harder pace for more reps. This week, we get a real opportunity to record a training best mile. Whilst it won't quite be a flat out run, it will be at a high enough level of effort to be counted as a reference time. Remember during the recovery periods, keep the legs moving, bring the breathing rate back down and keep an eye on the time! Divide you mile time by 4 to get your pace per 400m for the remaining runs, then aim to match or beat it. The 800m and 400m runs in particular should be noticeably quicker.

WEEK 9
DAY 2
WATCH USING QR CODE ON PAGE 54 ▶▶

WARM UP
5 X
- 3 BURPEES
- 3 WALKOUT TO UPDOG
- 5 KANG SQUATS

THE SESSION
3 X
- MAX FLOOR PRESS
- 15 UPRIGHT ROWS
- MAX PUSH PRESS
- 15 BENT OVER ROWS

16 MINUTE AMRAP
- 8 PUSH-UPS
- 16 STATIC LUNGES
- 8 BENCH DIPS
- 16 AIR SQUATS

COOL DOWN
- 1 MINUTE GROIN STRETCH
- 1 MINUTE CRUCIFIX

A change to the approach this week with the strength work, as we go to maximum on two movements; the floor press and the push press. It is important to note that we go to the limit of good form, not as many reps as we can physically manage. A mid-length conditioning workout forms the second part of the session. You most likely won't move non-stop, but the key is to minimise the rest periods and, when you do break, to keep it as short as possible. Although the movements are simple, and we are against the clock, form should remain the priority.

WEEK 9
DAY 3
WATCH USING QR CODE ON PAGE 54 ▶▶

WARM UP
3 X
- RUN 200M
- 30M HIGH KNEES
- 30M HEEL FLICKS
- 30M RUN HARD

THE SESSION
5-7 X 150M HILL REPS
- USE THE SAME HILL AS PREVIOUSLY IF AT ALL POSSIBLE
- FROM THE BOTTOM, RUN HARD UP, THEN TURN AROUND AND JOG BACK DOWN
- AT THE BOTTOM, IMMEDIATELY BEGIN THE NEXT RUN
- AFTER THE FINAL RUN, JOG/WALK BACK TO STRETCH
- TIME EACH REP, BUT DON'T WORRY ABOUT THE JOGS BACK DOWN
- PERFORM ONE MORE REP THAN LAST TIME, TRYING TO EQUAL OR BEAT PREVIOUS TIMES

COOL DOWN
- 1 MINUTE BAND OR STRAP HAMSTRING STRETCH
- 1 MINUTE SADDLE
- 30 SECONDS SPRINT CALF STRETCH

Hill reps plus one! We simply take the result from the last hill rep session, replicate all details, but add one more rep to the mix. Remember to try not to walk at all, but instead jog as slowly as you like to the bottom of the hill each time. Keep track of your times up the hill for reference.

WEEK 9
DAY 4
WATCH USING QR CODE ON PAGE 54 ▶▶

WARM UP
- 5-10 MINUTES OF WALK/RUN AT A STEADY PACE.
- TOWARDS THE END, INCREASE PACE TO THE PACE YOU'RE GOING TO USE FOR THE SESSION AND INCORPORATE TOE SWEEPS AND HIGH KNEES

THE SESSION
RUN FOR 30 MINUTES
- THIS IS A RECOVERY RUN, AND SHOULD BE PERFORMED AT 50-60% EFFORT
- SOME WALKING IS OKAY, BUT KEEP IT TO A MINIMUM
- IF YOU TRY TO IMPROVE ANYTHING OVER PREVIOUS WEEKS, REDUCE WALKING RATHER THAN INCREASING RUNNING PACE
- THIS SHOULD BE ON THE TRAIL IF POSSIBLE

COOL DOWN
- 1 MINUTE DEEP BAND/STRAP HAMSTRING STRETCH
- 1 MINUTE COSSACK

This is the same as last week. Avoid the urge to want to run further, or choose a harder route. If anything, walk less, however keep that running intensity low. As always with the trails, the more scenic it is, the more you can relax and enjoy it.

9 COMPLETE
THREE QUARTERS

Three quarters of the way through probably feels a little surreal. You have probably already forgotten what it feels like not to train every other day. This is the point at which working out becomes a fixture in your routine, a non-negotiable in your life. That's exactly what we need, for it to be a crutch, something you turn to to fix a bad day, or set you up for a productive one. Use fitness to enhance your life, and enable you to do more of what you love, rather than viewing it as a chore. Sure, you won't always feel like working out, but you will always be grateful for what working out allows you to do. Take a second to wrap that frame around your thoughts before each session, and hopefully you'll begin to view even the most difficult sessions in a positive light.

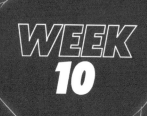

**SCAN FOR
VIDEO TUTORIAL**

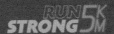

WEEK 10
DAY 1
WATCH USING QR CODE ON PAGE 60 ▶▶

WARM UP
- 5-10 MINUTES OF WALK/RUN AT A STEADY PACE.
- TOWARDS THE END, INCREASE PACE TO THE PACE YOU'RE GOING TO USE FOR THE SESSION AND INCORPORATE SHORT SPRINTS AND TURNS

THE SESSION
RUN: 2400M, 1600M, 800M
- TIME EACH RUN
- REST HALF THE TIME OF THE PREVIOUS RUN BEFORE RUNNING AGAIN
- RUN THE FIRST 2400M (1.5 MILES) AT ALMOST BEST EFFORT TO ESTABLISH A TIME (LOG THIS AS 1.5 MILE RECORD)
- DIVIDE THE 2400M TIME BY 3 TO GET YOU PACE PER 800M
- FOR THE REMAINDER OF THE RUNS, AIM TO MATCH OR BEAT THE 800M PACE OF THE FIRST RUN

COOL DOWN
- WALK FOR 3-5 MINUTES AFTER FINISHING THE LAST RUN
- STRETCH THE HAMSTRINGS AND CALVES AS REQUIRED

A double step forward this week; we both increase distance (both total and each run), and we drop the rest! As daunting as this sounds, you are now more prepared for it than you realise! As a guide, step off for your 2400m run at about 80%. This will begin to feel harder as you get further into it, but hold on. If you can maintain this pace, you will set a strong time. From here, rest half the time of that run, before running the 1600m. This run will be the hardest of the session, so convince yourself that you can maintain the pace before you step off. Positive self talk will not only help you through this session, but will be great practice for your 5km!

TOM HUNT TRAINING

WEEK 10 DAY 2
WATCH USING QR CODE ON PAGE 60 ▸▸

WARM UP
- 10-9-8-7-6-5-4-3-2-1 BURPEES & SQUATS

3 X
- 2 WALKOUTS
- 10 CHEST OPENERS

THE SESSION
3 X
- 12 THRUSTERS
- 12 SUMO DEADLIFT HIGH PULLS
- 12 STRICT PRESS
- 12 SINGLE ARM ROWS

3 ROUNDS FOR TIME
- 20 BURPEES
- 30 BOX JUMPS
- RUN 400M

COOL DOWN
- 1 MINUTE COUCH STRETCH
- 1 MINUTE CRUCIFIX

This week sees some new movements, and higher reps in the workout. As always, be sure to use the video to help with good movement patterns, and to help you get the most from the workout, adapting it to suit. The slightly longer run in this week's conditioning piece might catch you out a little bit, but just remember all the work you've done so far to give you a confidence boost beforehand!

WEEK 10
DAY 3
WATCH USING QR CODE ON PAGE 60 ▶▶

WARM UP
3 X
- RUN 200M
- 30M HIGH KNEES
- 30M HEEL FLICKS
- 30M RUN HARD

THE SESSION
4-5 X 250M HILL REPS
- USE THE SAME HILL AS PREVIOUSLY IF AT ALL POSSIBLE, BUT FOR A GREATER DISTANCE
- FROM THE BOTTOM, RUN HARD UP, THEN TURN AROUND AND JOG BACK DOWN
- AT THE BOTTOM, IMMEDIATELY BEGIN THE NEXT RUN
- AFTER THE FINAL RUN, JOG/WALK BACK TO STRETCH
- TIME EACH REP, BUT DON'T WORRY ABOUT THE JOGS BACK DOWN
- PERFORM A MINIMUM OF 4, BUT 5 IF YOU CAN MAINTAIN PACE

COOL DOWN
- 1 MINUTE KERB CALF STRETCH
- 1 MINUTE SADDLE
- 30 SECONDS SPRINT CALF STRETCH

Hill reps just got super-sized! We're going to take the same hill you have already used (if that's possible) and run an extra 100m up each time, making 250m total. The good news is that we're going less times, and the longer climb, means a longer recovery jog! Rules about not walking, and recovery jogging back to the bottom remain the same. This one is great for testing and building your mettle.

WEEK 10
DAY 4
WATCH USING QR CODE ON PAGE 60 ▶▶

WARM UP
- 5-10 MINUTES OF WALK/RUN AT A STEADY PACE.
- TOWARDS THE END, INCREASE PACE TO THE PACE YOU'RE GOING TO USE FOR THE SESSION AND INCORPORATE TOE SWEEPS AND HIGH KNEES

THE SESSION
RUN FOR 35 MINUTES
- THIS IS A RECOVERY RUN, AND SHOULD BE PERFORMED AT 50-60% EFFORT
- SOME WALKING IS OKAY, BUT KEEP IT TO A MINIMUM
- THE ONLY CHANGE FROM LAST WEEK SHOULD BE AN ADDITIONAL 5 MINUTES
- THIS SHOULD BE ON THE TRAIL IF POSSIBLE

COOL DOWN
- 1 MINUTE DEEP BAND/STRAP HAMSTRING STRETCH
- 1 MINUTE COSSACK

We're adding 5 minutes to your trail run this week, but other than that, the objective remains the same. Steady running, with the ability to answer in short sentences throughout. Keep walking to a minimum, and avoid the temptation to speed up if it feels good. Try a new route and some new views if it's convenient. Mixing up your route, your surroundings, and your views on these slower runs can be great for the soul, and even serve as motivation if you pick the right places

10 COMPLETE
THE LAST 'NORMAL' WEEK IS DONE!

Normal might be an odd choice of wording, but chances are, training is probably becoming quite normal for you now. It might be almost odd to think of changing your routine, but I can assure you, it will be short lived. Heading into week 11, volume and intensity drop back, and in week 12 we see the final challenge, but it's important to remember that your final 5km run isn't the end, but merely a waypoint on your route. Why am I taking time to talk about this with two weeks left to go? Because this knowledge will help you approach the next two weeks with the right mindset; one of reflection and assessment, rather than pass or fail.

WEEK 11

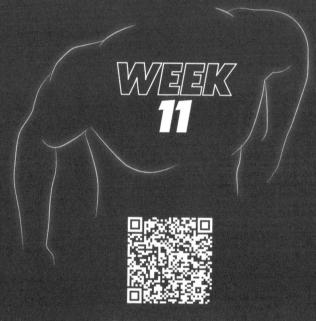

SCAN FOR VIDEO TUTORIAL

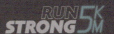

WEEK 11
DAY 1
WATCH USING QR CODE ON PAGE 66 ▶▶

WARM UP
- 5-10 MINUTES OF WALK/RUN AT A STEADY PACE.
- TOWARDS THE END, INCREASE PACE TO THE PACE YOU'RE GOING TO USE FOR THE SESSION AND INCORPORATE SHORT SPRINTS AND TURNS

THE SESSION
RUN: 3000M, 2000M
- TIME EACH RUN
- REST THE HALF THE TIME AS THE PREVIOUS RUN BEFORE RUNNING AGAIN
- RUN THE 3000M AT 80-90%, THEN MAKE SURE YOU SET A FASTER PACE ON THE 2KM
- REALLY FOCUS ON BREATHING THROUGHOUT THE REST PERIOD, KEEPING THE LEGS MOVING AND THE ARMS DOWN

COOL DOWN
- WALK FOR 3-5 MINUTES AFTER FINISHING THE LAST RUN
- STRETCH THE HAMSTRINGS AND CALVES AS REQUIRED

A bit of a pacing test for next week. The lesson to be learned here is running a little quicker towards the end of the session. This run is the same distance as the 5k you have trained for, at almost the same pace, but with a little rest after the first 3km. Use the final 2km to get used to running at the pace you plan on running your 5km next week. If possible, use the 5km route you have planned as a bit of a test run, and to make yourself aware of any little hills, sharp turns, road crossings, or indeed anything that might help.

WEEK 11
DAY 2

WATCH USING QR CODE ON PAGE 66 ▶▶

WARM UP
5 X
- 5 BURPEES
- 3 WALKOUTS
- 5 KANG SQUATS
- 10 EMPTY PRESSES

THE SESSION
3 X
- 15 THRUSTERS
- 15 SUMO DEADLIFT HIGH PULLS
- 15 STRICT PRESS
- 15 SINGLE ARM ROWS

5 ROUNDS FOR TIME
- 30 MOUNTAIN CLIMBERS
- 20 GOBLET SQUATS
- 10 BROAD JUMPS
- 5 REVERSE BURPEES

COOL DOWN
- 1 MINUTE COUCH STRETCH
- 1 MINUTE CRUCIFIX

Some familiar, well worn movements, and some new twists. Some of these are tough to describe, so take an extra few minutes with the video for this one, and really work on form, and speed. This is a near sprint workout, and should be relatively short, in spite of how it might look. Set aside a solid hour for the session though, as once we factor in the strength work, this is a decent workout. It's also the last big session you will do before your final 5km, so make the most of it!

WEEK 11
DAY 3
WATCH USING QR CODE ON PAGE 66 ▸▸

WARM UP
3 X
- RUN 200M
- 30M HIGH KNEES
- 30M HEEL FLICKS
- 30M RUN HARD

THE SESSION
RUN 5KM
- AIM TO NOT WALK
- DO NOT RACE, BE CONSERVATIVE WITH YOUR PACE
- IF YOU FIND YOURSELF STRUGGLING, SLOW DOWN YOUR RUNNING AND FOCUS ON YOUR BREATH
- WORK BETWEEN 70-80% EFFORT THROUGHOUT
- AVOID THE TEMPTATION TO SPEED UP TOWARDS THE END

COOL DOWN
- 1 MINUTE KERB CALF STRETCH
- 1 MINUTE SADDLE
- 30 SECONDS SPRINT CALF STRETCH

We're winding it right back today. This 5km serves two purposes; a little confidence booster so you know the distance isn't a problem next week, it's just about how quickly you can move, and secondly it's a nice opportunity to shake the legs out and loosen off. It might be worth taking an extra few minutes to top those stretches up after his one, and schedule a long soak in the bath afterwards. Remember to select a flat, quiet route, on concrete. A different route to the one you have planned for the final 5km is okay today, but if your selection is limited, doing the same one won't hurt.

11 COMPLETE
YOU'RE READY!

You might not feel it, but you are. If you're nervous about taking on your 5km time trial, that's pretty normal, but it's likely you're at least partly excited too! Probably the best way to add some perspective is this; what would have happened if you attempted this 12 weeks ago? So unless something has gone very wrong, you're going to be in a better place than you were then, and that's all you're checking! Whatever your result, it serves as a starting point for the next part of your journey. So with that in mind, definitely give it your all, but try and enjoy it, and be proud of how far you've come too!

WEEK 12

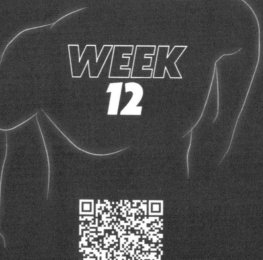

SCAN FOR VIDEO TUTORIAL

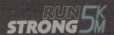

WEEK 12
DAY 1
WATCH USING QR CODE ON PAGE 72 ▶▶

WARM UP
- 5-10 MINUTES OF WALK/RUN AT A STEADY PACE.
- TOWARDS THE END, INCREASE PACE TO THE PACE YOU'RE GOING TO USE FOR THE SESSION AND INCORPORATE SHORT SPRINTS AND TURNS.
- AS A MINIMUM, COVER 400-500M IN 100-200M BURSTS AT THE PACE YOU PLAN ON USING.
- BE SLIGHTLY BREATHLESS, SWEATY AND WITH AN ELEVATED HEART RATE WHEN YOU BEGIN

THE SESSION
RUN: 3000M, 2000M
- SET OFF AT THE PACE YOU USED FOR THE FINAL 2KM LAST WEEK
- PREPARE MENTALLY FOR THE 3RD AND 4TH KM BEING PARTICULARLY TOUGH. YOU CAN RUN THROUGH THAT DISCOMFORT, BUT YOU NEED TO BE READY TO DO SO.
- FOR THAT FINAL KM, YOU HAVE NOTHING TO LOSE. EARN YOUR FINISH TIME AND POST YOURSELF A RECORD TO GET AFTER IN THE FUTURE.
- SET UP FOR SUCCESS; KNOW YOUR ROUTE, HAVE YOUR WATCH READY, STAY HYDRATED BEFOREHAND, AND DON'T SET OFF TOO FAST!
- YOU'VE GOT THIS, NOW GO AND ENJOY THE RESULTS OF YOUR EFFORTS!

COOL DOWN
- WALK FOR 3-5 MINUTES AFTER FINISHING THE LAST RUN
- STRETCH THE HAMSTRINGS AND CALVES AS REQUIRED

Here we are! It's easy to get nervous and make this into something bigger than it needs to be. Try looking at it this way, you have EARNED today. All the hard work you have done has allowed you to not only take on this run, but to push yourself and get a time in the books that you know is your best effort. That in itself is something to be hugely proud of. Not many people see challenges through, you have, and that's awesome!

TOM HUNT TRAINING

WEEK 12
DAY 2
WATCH USING QR CODE BELOW ▶▶

THE SESSION
ONLINE STRETCH FLOW
- LOG INTO THE WATCH LINK USING THE QR CODE BELOW TO FOLLOW ALONG.

SCAN FOR VIDEO TUTORIAL

This flow is repeated from earlier in the programme. Take it easy, relax into it, and see if you notice positions that are any easier or harder than last time!

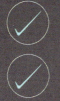

12 COMPLETE
CONGRATULATIONS!

THANK YOU

From me, but also from your body, thank you! Why from me? Because you have put your faith in a different way of approaching this particular challenge, and taken a shot at my method. Although I have used and honed this approach with many people from all walks of life over the years, this is the first time I have taken stock, and put my methods into a coherent plan on paper. Why from your body? Because you're now fitter and healthier than you were 12 weeks ago, and likely happier too! I don't mean you'll be walking around with a permanent grin, but I do mean your energy levels will be higher, daily tasks will have become easier, and your mental resilience has been upgraded. That makes for a happier, more fulfilling life.

WHAT'S NEXT?

Well that depends on you. If this was your first foray into running, and you're still over the 30 minute mark for your 5km, the one option would be to do this programme again. Whilst repeating might not sound like much fun, or may even sound like defeat, it is far from it. Firstly, it's valuable to revisit sessions, and not improvements; not only in time, pace or distance, but also in recovery, levels of discomfort and attitude. These are areas often overlooked when we assess progress. Secondly, the programme will be a different one a second time through. You are in a very different place to 12 weeks ago, so your results will be different, allowing you to get new and different benefits from the programme. I would suggest only running this programme twice through before moving on though, as the returns will diminish beyond that.

If you have managed to get a time that you're happy with, and want to take the momentum forward into a new challenge, then i would suggest Run Strong Volume 2 - 10km. This has an entry suggestion of a sub 30 minute 5km time, but will work for anyone who can run 5km without stopping, and benefit those who are much quicker too. In addition to adding distance to your arsenal, this programme will make you quicker too! The 12 weeks begins by building a distance base, then culminates by targeting your speed and speed endurance. Visit www.tomhunttraining.com/shop to find the latest eBook releases, or www.tomhunttraining.com to see the full selection of online programmes available to follow.

If you used this programme to get moving again after an injury, or time away from training, maybe you progressed quickly through this, and want something a little more extreme? From half-marathons, marathons and ultra marathons, to strength sports, obstacle course races and general fitness, there is a programme, or a bespoke option to suit you at www.tomhunttraining.com If you don't see what you want right away, then feel free to send a message to enquire in detail.

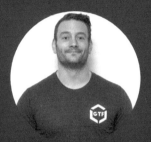

ABOUT THE AUTHOR

Tom Hunt has spent the majority of his life as a soldier in the British Army, completing almost 13 years as a regular soldier, and he is currently approaching 5 years in the Army Reserve. In 2011, whilst responsible for training new recruits, he found the long hours and demanding schedule, combined with other personal factors, led to him becoming the unhealthiest and least fit version of himself to date. He discovered health, fitness and rediscovered sports, and has since never looked back.

Since embarking on a journey towards a healthier and fitter lifestyle, Tom has also found a passion for self-experimentation and extreme challenges. Tom has completed numerous half-marathons, marathons, one and two day ultra marathons, a relay ultra marathon and a mountain iron distance triathlon. This summer, he completed a 50 mile run wearing a 20lb weight vest, and is currently training to set a Guinness World Record for distance covered in 24 hours, carrying 40lb.

In addition to endurance and ultra endurance events, Tom has competed in and coaches weightlifting, strongman, CrossFit®, triathlon and a wide variety of sports.

Tom is currently the Head Coach and owner at GT Fitness, and GTF Barbell Club, in Uttoxeter, is a coach for the Army Weightlifting Team, and is a Physical Training Instructor and military instructor for the Army Reserve, working with students and potential officers.

RUN 5K
STRONG 5M

Published by Active Athlete Limited
© 2020 Stafford
All rights reserved. No part of this book may be reproduced or modified in any form, including photocopying, recording, or by any information storage and retrieval system, without permission in writing from the publisher.

**TOM HUNT
TRAINING**

Printed in Great Britain
by Amazon

GLOUCESTE AND BRIS

A GENEALOGICAL BIBLIOGRAPHY

— BY —
STUART RAYMOND

FEDERATION OF FAMILY HISTORY SOCIETIES

Published by the
Federation of Family History Societies,
c/o The Benson Room, Birmingham & Midland Institute,
Margaret Street, Birmingham B3 3BS, England.

Copies also obtainable from:
S.A. & M.J. Raymond, 6 Russet Avenue, Exeter EX1 3QB, England.
S.A. & M.J. Raymond, P.O. Box 255, Belmont, Vic. 3216, Australia.

Copyright © S.A. Raymond, 1992

Typesetting from computer disks and layout by Stuart Raymond and Jeremy Gibson.
Printed by Parchment (Oxford) Limited.

Cataloguing in publication data:

Raymond, Stuart A., 1945-
Gloucestershire and Bristol: a genealogical bibliography.
British genealogical bibliographies.
Birmingham, England: Federation of Family History Societies, 1992.

DDC 016.9291094241

ISBN 1 872094 34 1

ISSN: 1033-2065

CONTENTS

Page

Introduction ... 4
Libraries and Record Offices ... 5
Abbreviations ... 5
1. The History of Gloucestershire and Bristol ... 7
2. Bibliography and Archives ... 9
3. Journals and Newspapers ... 12
4. Names and Dialect ... 13
5. Biographical Dictionaries, Genealogical Directories, and Occupational Lists ... 13
6. Visitation Returns and Heraldry ... 18
7. Family Histories ... 20
8. Parish Registers and other records of Births, Marriages and Deaths ... 33
9. Probate Records and *Inquisitions Post Mortem* ... 43
10. Monumental Inscriptions ... 48
11. Official Lists of Names ... 54
12. Directories and Maps ... 57
13. Religious Records ... 59
14. Estate and Family Papers ... 63
15. National, County and Local Administration ... 70
16. Education ... 74
17. Emigration ... 75
Family Name Index ... 76
Place Name Index ... 79
Author Index ... 84

INTRODUCTION

This bibliography is intended primarily for genealogists. It is, however, hoped that it will also prove useful to historians, librarians, research students, and anyone else interested in Bristol and Gloucestershire history and families. It is intended to be used in conjunction with my *English genealogy: an introductory bibliography*, and the other titles in the *British genealogical bibliographies* series. A full list of these titles is given on the back cover.

Many genealogists, when they begin their research, fail to realise just how much information has been published, and is readily available in printed form. Not infrequently, they head straight for the archives, when they would probably do best to check printed sources first. When faced with the vast array of tomes possessed by major reference libraries, they do not know where to begin. This bibliography, in conjunction with the others in the series, is intended to help you find that beginning, and to provide guidance in following through the quest for ancestors. My aim has been to list everything relating to Gloucestershire and Bristol that has been published, and is likely to be of use to genealogists. In general, I have not included works which are national in scope, but which have local content. Such works may be identified in *English genealogy: an introductory bibliography*. I have also excluded the innumerable notes and queries found in such journals as *G.N.Q.*, and *J.B.A.*, except where the content is of importance. Where I have included such notes, replies to them are cited in the form 'see also', with no reference to the names of respondents. Local and church histories have also been excluded, except in a few cases. Such histories are frequently invaluable for genealogical purposes, but a full listing of them would require another volume.

Be warned – I cannot claim that this bibliography is comprehensive. Neither do I claim that it is totally accurate. Some works have been deliberately excluded; others I have undoubtedly missed. If you come across anything I have missed, please let me know, so that it can be included in a second edition in due course.

Most works listed here are readily available in the libraries listed below – although no library holds everything. Even if you are overseas, you should be able to find copies of the more important reference works in larger research libraries. However, some items may prove difficult to locate – particularly articles in local periodicals. Never fear! Librarians believe in the doctrine of the universal availability of publications, and most public libraries are able to tap into the international interlibrary loans system. Your local library should be able to borrow most of the items listed here, even if it has to go overseas to obtain them.

The work of compiling this bibliography has depended heavily on the resources of the libraries I have used. These included Bristol Reference Library, Bristol University Library, Gloucester City Library, Exeter City Library, Exeter University Library, and the Devon and Exeter Institution. I have also borrowed material by post from the Yorkshire Archaeological Society, the Somerset and Dorset Family History Society, and Devon Family History Society. I am grateful to the librarians of all these institutions for their help. I am also grateful to Cynthia Hanson, Stella Pugh, and Terry Humphries, who typed this book, to Brian Christmas for proof-reading it, and to Jeremy Gibson, for seeing it through the press and providing much needed encouragement.

Stuart A. Raymond.

LIBRARIES AND RECORD OFFICES

The major libraries and record offices concerned with Gloucestershire and Bristol history are:

Gloucestershire County Library,
Shire Hall, Quayside Wing,
GLOUCESTER GL1 2HY.

Gloucestershire Record Office,
Worcester Street,
GLOUCESTER GL1 3DW.

Bristol Central Library,
College Green,
BRISTOL BS1 5TL.

Bristol Record Office,
B Bond Warehouse, Smeaton Road,
BRISTOL BS1 6XN.

Bristol University Library,
Tyndall Avenue,
BRISTOL BS8 1TJ.

In addition, most branches of Gloucestershire County Library hold local studies material.

BIBLIOGRAPHIC PRESENTATION

Authors' names are in SMALL CAPITALS. Book and journal titles are in *italics*. Articles appearing in journals and material, such as parish register transcripts, forming only part of books are in inverted commas and textface type. Volume numbers are in **bold** and the individual number of the journal may be shown in parentheses. These are normally followed by the place of publication (except where this is London, which is omitted), the name of the publisher and the date of publication. In the case of articles, further figures indicate page numbers.

ABBREVIATIONS

B.G.A.S.Tr.	*Bristol and Gloucestershire Archaeological Society Transactions.*
C.K.L.H.S.B.	*Charlton Kings Local History Society Bulletin.*
G.N.Q.	*Gloucestershire Notes and Queries.*
G.P.R.M.	PHILLIMORE, W.P.W. *Gloucestershire Parish Registers: Marriages.*
J.B.A.	*Journal of the Bristol and Avon Family History Society.*
J.G.F.H.S.	*Journal of the Gloucestershire Family History Society.*
M.G.H.	*Miscellanea Genealogica et Heraldica.*
P.P.R.S.	*Phillimore's Parish Register Series*

1. THE HISTORY OF GLOUCESTERSHIRE AND BRISTOL

How did your ancestors live, work eat and sleep? What was the world they lived in like? If you want to know the answers to questions like this, and to understand the world of parish registers, estate surveys, and subsidy rolls, you need to read up on local history. For Gloucestershire, a good beginning is provided by:
SMITH, B.S., & RALPH, E. *History of Bristol and Gloucestershire*. Henley: Darwen Finlayson, 1972.
The authoritative work, still not complete, is:
The Victoria history of the county of Gloucester. Archibald Constable, 1907- . Contents: **2**. Ecclesiastical history. **4**. The city of Gloucester. **6**. Slaughter Hundred; Tewkesbury Hundred, upper division; Westminster Hundred, upper division. **7**. Brightwells Barrow and Ramsgate Hundreds. **8**. Cleeve Hundred; Deerhurst Hundred; Tewkesbury Hundred, lower division; Tibblestone Hundred; Westminster Hundred, lower division. **10**. Westbury and Whitstone Hundreds. **11**. Bisley and Longtree Hundreds.
Other interesting general works include:
FINBERG, H.P.R., ed. *Gloucestershire studies*. Leicester: Leicester University Press, 1957.
FINBERG, H.P.R. *The Gloucestershire landscape*. Making of the English landscape series. Hodder & Stoughton, 1975.
FINBERG, JOSCELINE. *The Cotswolds*. Eyre Methuen, 1977.
HADFIELD, CHARLES & ALICE MARY, eds. *The Cotswolds: a new study*. Newton Abbot: David & Charles, 1973.
MACINNES, C.M., & WHITTARD, W.F, ed. *Bristol and its adjoining counties*. Bristol: [ ], 1955. Reprinted East Ardsley: E.P. Publishing, 1973.
WALKER, FRANK. *The Bristol region*. Nelson, 1972.

For Bristol, many valuable historical works have been published in:
Local history pamphlets. Bristol: Historical Association, Bristol Branch, c.1962-
Particular periods are dealt with in:
HILTON, R.H. *A medieval society: the West Midlands at the end of the thirteenth century*. Weidenfeld & Nicolson, 1966.
SAUL, NIGEL. *Knights and esquires: the Gloucestershire gentry in the fourteenth century*. Oxford: Clarendon, 1981.
JOHNSON, JOAN. *Tudor Gloucestershire*. Gloucester: Alan Sutton and Gloucestershire County Library, 1985.
SHARP, BUCHANAN. *In contempt of all authority; rural artisans and riot in the West of England, 1586-1660*. Berkeley: University of California Press, 1980. Mainly concerned with Gloucestershire and Wiltshire.
JOHNSON, JOAN. *The Gloucestershire gentry*. Gloucester: Alan Sutton, 1989. General survey, 16-19th c.
A useful collection of documents typical of those the local historian – and the genealogist – can expect to encounter is provided by:
WHERRY, ANTHONY. *Four hundred years of Gloucestershire life*. [Cheltenham?]: Historical Association, Cheltenham & District Branch, 1971.

The historical uses of genealogical sources are demonstrated in a number of works:
JORDAN, W.K. *The forming of the charitable institutions of the West of England: a study of the changing pattern of social aspirations in Bristol and Somerset, 1480-1660*. Transactions of the American Philosophical Society, N.S., **50**(8), 1-99. Based on wills.
PORTER, STEPHEN. 'Age at baptism in Gloucester in the mid seventeenth century', *B.G.A.S.Tr.* **90**, 1980, 131-4.
RIPLEY, PETER. 'Village and town: occupations and wealth in the hinterland of Gloucester, 1660-1700', *Agricultural history review*, **32**(2), 1984, 170-8. Based on probate records.
RIPLEY, PETER. 'The economy of the city of Gloucester, 1660-1740', *B.G.A.S.Tr.* **98**, 1980, 135-53. Based on probate inventories, which are listed.
ROLLISON, D. 'Property, ideology and popular culture in a Gloucestershire village, 1660-1740', *Past & Present* **93**, 1981, 107-97. Includes list of persons active in the 'groaning' at Weston Birt in 1716, giving ages, occupations and residence. Fascinating!
WHITING, J.R.S. *Prison reform in Gloucestershire, 1776-1820: a study of the work of Sir George Onesiphorus Paul, Bart*. Phillimore, 1975. The list of original sources provides many potential leads.
WOODS, S.R. 'Shirehampton: the 1851 census', *B.G.A.S.Tr.* **89**, 1970, 145-55.

History of Gloucestershire and Bristol continued

The earliest major works on Gloucestershire history were originally published in the eighteenth century, and have recently been re-printed. All three incorporate parochial surveys, and contain much material of genealogical value:

ATKYNS, SIR ROBERT. *The ancient and present state of Gloucestershire.* East Ardsley: EP Publishing, 1974. Originally published W. Bowyer, 1712.

RUDDER, SAMUEL. *A new history of Gloucestershire.* Dursley: Alan Sutton, 1977. Originally published Cirencester: the author, 1779. Includes many monumental inscriptions, Domesday book *etc.*

BIGLAND, RALPH. *Historical, monumental and genealogical collections relative to the county of Gloucester.* Gloucestershire Record series, 2- . Gloucester: B.G.A.S., 1989- . Pt. 1. Abbenhall-Cromhall. Pt. 2. Daglingworth-Moreton Valence. Pts. 3 and 4 not yet published. Originally published in 2 vols, John Nicholls, 1791. For the heraldry in this work, see F. Were, 'Index to the heraldry in Bigland's *History of Gloucestershire*', *B.G.A.S.Tr.* **28**, 1905, 147-50.

Atkins' work was corrected in:

FOSBROOKE, THOMAS DUDLEY. *Abstracts of records and manuscripts respecting the county of Gloucester, formed into a history, correcting very erroneous accounts, and supplying numerous deficiencies, in Sir Rob. Atkins and subsequent writers.* 2 vols. Gloucester: Jos. Harris, 1807. Parochial survey arranged by hundred; includes many pedigrees.

For Gloucester, Bigland's history was continued in:

FOSBROOKE, THOMAS DUDLEY. *An original history of the city of Gloucester almost wholly compiled from new materials ... including also the original papers of the late Ralph Bigland ...* John Nichols & Sons, 1819. Reprinted Gloucester: Alan Sutton, 1976. Includes notes on many monumental inscriptions.

See also:

RUDGE, THOMAS. *The history and antiquities of Gloucester, from the earliest period to the present time ...* Gloucester: J. Wood 1811. Includes lists of bishops, abbots and other dignitaries, with monumental inscriptions.

A useful genealogical guide to Gloucester is provided by:

PHELPS, G.F. 'Gloucester city and its parishes', *J.G.F.H.S.* **14**, 1982, 6-11.

For Bristol, see:

BARRETT, WILLIAM. *The history and antiquities of the city of Bristol.* Bristol: William Pine, 1789. Includes lists of surveyors, sheriffs, clergy, benefactors, monumental inscriptions etc.

See also:

LATIMER, JOHN. *The annals of Bristol in the seventeenth century.* Bristol: William George's Sons, 1900. Includes lists of civic dignitaries. Latimer wrote similar works dealing with the 16th, 18th and 19th centuries.

There are numerous other county and local histories of Gloucestershire, many of which have genealogical value. A few are listed in the appropriate chapter below, but a complete list would occupy at least another volume. The intention here is merely to whet the appetite; if you seek more information, consult the volumes listed in chapter 2.

2. BIBLIOGRAPHY AND ARCHIVES

A basic introductory bibliography on Gloucestershire history is provided by:
Neighbourhood search. Gloucester: Gloucestershire County Library, 1984.
Another useful introductory guide is:
SMITH, BRIAN S. *Gloucestershire local history handbook.* 2nd ed. Gloucester: Gloucestershire Community Council, 1975.
For Bristol and the southern part of the county, see:
MOORE, J.S., ed. *Avon local history handbook.* Chichester: Phillimore for Avon Local History Association, 1979.

The literature of Gloucestershire has provided work for many bibliographers. The earliest comprehensive work, still useful, was:
HYETT, FRANCIS ADAMS & BAZELEY, WILLIAM. *The bibliographer's manual of Gloucestershire literature, being a classified catalogue of books, pamphlets, broadsides and other printed matter relating to the county of Gloucester or city of Bristol.* 3 vols. Gloucester: J. Bellows, 1895-7.
The supplement to this manual is of particular value to genealogists, since it lists pedigrees, and includes many bibliographical notices:
HYETT, F.A. & AUSTIN, ROLAND. *Supplement to the bibliographer's manual of Gloucestershire literature, being a classified catalogue of bibliographical and genealogical literature relating to men and women connected by birth, office, or many years' residence, with the county of Gloucester or the city of Bristol, with descriptive and explanatory notes.* 2 vols. Gloucester: John Bellows, 1915-16.
The most useful Gloucestershire bibliography is:
AUSTIN, ROLAND. *Catalogue of the Gloucestershire collection: books, pamphlets and documents in the Gloucester Public Library relating to the county, cities, towns and villages of Gloucestershire.* Gloucester: Henry Osborne [for the Library], 1928.
Austin's catalogue lists the contents of the most important Gloucestershire collection, and includes manuscript material as well as books. Updates have not been published, but are available in the library. The catalogues of three other important collectors have also been published:
AUSTIN, ROLAND. *The Dancey gift: catalogue of manuscripts, books, pamphlets and prints relating to the City and County of Gloucester ... deposited in the Gloucester County Library.* [Gloucester]: Gloucester City Council, 1911.
AUSTIN, ROLAND. *Catalogue of Gloucestershire books collected by Sir Francis Hyett of Painswick and placed in the Shire Hall.* Gloucester: H. Osborne for Gloucestershire County Council, 1949.
Collectanea Glocestriensia, or, a catalogue of books, tracts, coins &c., relating to the county of Gloucester, in the possession of John Delafield Phelps esq., Chavenage House. William Nicol, 1842. Includes lists of portraits, with bibliographical notes.
For Bristol, a comprehensive bibliography is provided by:
MATHEWS, E.R. NORRIS. ed. *Bristol bibliography. City & county of Bristol municipal public libraries. A catalogue of the books, pamphlets, collectanea etc relating to Bristol, contained in the Central Reference Library.* Bristol: Libraries Committee, 1916.
Some more recent Bristol material of interest to genealogists is noted in:
DIXON, NICK. *An archaeological bibliography of Bristol.* Bristol: Bristol City Museum & Art Gallery, 1987.
Brief notes on rare Gloucestershire material at the Bodleian Library, Oxford, are provided by:
'Gloucestershire references in the Bodleian Library', *G.N.Q.* **6**, 1896, 117-20, 149-51, and 170-71; **7**, 1900, 81-83, 159-60, and 168-73.
The Gloucestershire content of three 19th century genealogical journals are noted in:
GENEALOGIST. 'Nichols' *Collectanea topographica et genealogica*', *G.N.Q.* **2**, 1884, 204-41.
GENEALOGIST. 'Nichols' *Herald & Genealogist*', *G.N.Q.* **2**, 1884, 191-2.
GENEALOGIST. 'Howard's *Miscellanea genealogica et heraldica*', *G.N.Q.* **2**, 1884, 212-3.

Archival material should not be consulted until you have checked all the relevant published works. When you have done this, consult:
RICHARDS, M.E. *Gloucestershire family history.* 2nd ed. Gloucester: Gloucestershire County Council, 1983. General discussion of archival sources.
Richards has also listed parish registers, monumental inscription transcripts, census microfilm *etc.*, held by the Gloucestershire Record Office:
RICHARDS, M.E. *Handlist of genealogical sources.* [Gloucester]: Gloucestershire Record Office, 1982. Includes parish registers, monumental inscriptions, 1851 census microfilm *etc.*

Bibliography and Archives continued

The main guide to the Gloucestershire Record Office is:
KINGSLEY, N.W. *Handlist of the contents of the Gloucestershire Record Office*. [Gloucester]: Gloucestershire County Council, 1988.
For accessions, see:
Gloucestershire: report of the Records Committee of the County Council 1936-1938. [Gloucester: the Committee], 1938. Subsequent reports cover 1939-40, 1941-45, 1945-51, 1952-68. All list accessions. Continued by:
GLOUCESTERSHIRE RECORD OFFICE. *Annual report*. Gloucester: the office, 1970-71.
An annual list of accessions was also published in: 'Gloucestershire Records Office: list of principal accessions, 19–', *B.G.A.S.Tr.* **68-97**, 1949-79.
A further decade is covered in:
KINGSLEY, NICHOLAS. 'Gloucestershire Record Office: summary of accessions, 1979-1988', *B.G.A.S.Tr.* **106**, 1988, 225-7.
The collections of Gloucestershire Record Office were originally based on the Quarter Sessions archives. These are separately listed:
GRAY, I.E., & GAYDON, A.T. *Gloucestershire quarter sessions archives, 1660-1889, and other official records: a descriptive catalogue*. Gloucester: Gloucestershire County Council, 1958. This is reviewed in:
GROOME, W.I. 'Gloucestershire quarter sessions archives, 1660-1889, and other records', *B.G.A.S.Tr.* **77**, 1958, 171-3.
See also:
Gloucestershire: a catalogue of county records and of the most important books and documents relating to county administration in the custody of the Clerk of the Peace and Clerk of the County Council of Gloucestershire, and also of the record publications in the library, Shire Hall, Gloucester. Gloucester: Chave & Bland, 1898. Brief list.
Report of the Committee appointed to supervise the rearrangement of the records, books and documents in the Shire Hall. Gloucester: Gloucestershire Standing Joint Committee, 1897. Mainly a catalogue of county records.
The Gloucestershire Record Office, 1936-1986: a short history ... Gloucester: the Office, 1986. Brief pamphlet, general background.
GRAY, IRVINE E., 'Local archives of Great Britain, XXV: the Gloucestershire Records Office', *Archives*, **6**, 1963-64, 178-85.
MANSFIELD, GWEN. 'Gloucestershire County Records Office ... : guide to contents (rough jottings)', *J.G.F.H.S.* **6**, 1980, 15-16.

SMITH, B.S. 'Sources for genealogy in the Gloucestershire Record Office', *J.B.A.* **4**, 1976, 20-22. Brief note.
SMITH, BRIAN. 'Gloucestershire Record Office', *Journal of the Society of Archivists* **6**, 1978-81, 99. Brief description of new office.
'Record Office review: steady improvement', *Family tree magazine* **1**(2), 1985, 22. Account of Gloucestershire Record Office.

The contents of the Bristol Archives Office are listed in:
RALPH, ELIZABETH. *Guide to the Bristol Archives Office, city and county of Bristol*. Bristol: Bristol Corporation, 1971.
More recent accessions are listed in two works:
'Bristol Archives Office: principal accessions, 19–', *B.G.A.S.Tr.* **91-7**, 1972-9, *passim*.
City of Bristol Record Office, 1974-1983: report of the city archivist. Bristol: City Archivist, 1983.
See also:
BRISTOL RECORD OFFICE. *Sources for the family historian*. Information leaflet **1**. Bristol: the office, 1986.
RALPH, ELIZABETH & MASTERS, BETTY. 'Local archives of Great Britain XIV: the City of Bristol Record Office', *Archives* **3**, 1957-8, 88-96.
ROBERTS, GEOFF. 'Bristol Record Office', *J.B.A.*, **2**, **3**, 1981, 11-12. Brief discussion.
HARDING, N. DERMOTT. 'Treasures of the Corporation of Bristol', *Apollo* **5**, 1927, 235-43. Description of treasures from the archives.
BRISTOL RECORD OFFICE. *Sources for the history of buildings*. Information leaflet **3**. Bristol: the office, 1987.

Some important manuscript material is also held by Gloucester City Library. See:
WOODMAN, V.A. 'Local archives of Great Britain, XXVI: archives in the Gloucester City Library', *Archives* **6**, 1963-4, 225-8.
Gloucester City Libraries: local history manuscript collection and regulations. Local history pamphlet **1**. Rev. ed. [Gloucester]: Gloucester City Libraries, c.1968. Brief description of collections, including diocesan records, Hockaday abstracts of Gloucestershire records, Smyth of Nibley papers *etc*.

Bibliography and Archives continued

Records relating to the Gloucestershire parishes. Local history pamphlet **3**. Gloucester: City Libraries, 1960. Index to collections in the City Library, including Hockaday abstracts, bishops transcripts, terriers, deeds, tithe maps *etc.* Amongst the papers at Gloucester City Library are the papers of John Smyth of Nibley, the seventeenth century antiquary. These relate to the Berkeley family, the Hundred of Berkeley, and to local government and manorial administration. See:

Smyth of Nibley papers. Local history sources **1**. Gloucester County Library, 1978.

HAINES, ROBERT J. 'The Smyth of Nibley papers', *J.G.F.H.S.* **15**, 1982, 7-10.

LINDLEY, E.S. 'A John Smyth bibliography', *B.G.A.S.Tr.* **80**, 1961, 121-31.

A number of publications deal with the archives of the dioceses of Gloucester and Bristol:

KIRBY, ISOBEL M. *Diocese of Bristol: a catalogue of the records of the bishops and archdeacons and of the dean and chapter.* Bristol: Bristol Corporation, 1970.

KIRBY, ISOBEL M. *Diocese of Gloucester: A catalogue of the records of the bishop and archdeacons.* Records of the diocese of Gloucester, **1**. Gloucester: Gloucester City Corporation, 1968.

KIRBY, ISOBEL M. *Diocese of Gloucester: a catalogue of the records of the dean and chapter, including the former St Peter's Abbey.* Records of the Diocese of Gloucester, **2**. Gloucester: Gloucestershire County Council, 1967.

KIRBY, ISOBEL. 'Gloucester Diocesan records', *B.G.A.S.Tr.* **87**, 1968, 119-30. General discussion of archives.

MACRAY, W.D. 'Records of the Diocese of Gloucester', in HISTORICAL MANUSCRIPTS COMMISSION. *Report on manuscripts in various collections* **7**. Cd. 6722. H.M.S.O., 1914, 44-69.

HOCKADAY, F.S. 'Gloucester diocesan records', *Gloucester diocesan magazine* **7**, 1912, 151-6 and 188-91; **8**, 1913, 55-6, 69-71, 108-11 and 142-6; **9**, 1914, 30-1, 48-9, 82-4 and 131-2; **10**, 1915, 30-2. Not completed.

AUSTIN, ROLAND. 'The late Mr F.S. Hockaday and the records of the Diocese', *Gloucester diocesan magazine*, 1924, 116-7. Brief discussion of Hockaday's work.

For the archives of the Roman Catholic Diocese of Clifton, which includes Gloucestershire, Wiltshire and Somerset, see:

CLOSE, JUDITH. 'The archives of the Diocese of Clifton', *South Western Catholic History* **1**, 1983, 3-9.

BRADLEY, ANNE. 'Interim report on Clifton Diocesan archives deposited at Bristol Records Office', *South Western Catholic History* **4**, 1986, 6-11. Includes list of registers.

If your ancestors were involved in business, it may be useful to consult:

GREEN, JENNIFER, OLLERENSHAW, PHILIP & WARDLEY, PETER. *Business in Avon and Somerset: a survey of archives.* Bristol: Bristol Polytechnic, 1991.

Gloucestershire manuscripts in the British Library (formerly the British Museum) are listed in:

HYETT, F.A. 'A catalogue of manuscripts in the British Museum relating to the county of Gloucester and the city of Bristol', *B.G.A.S.Tr.* **20**, 1895-7, 161-221.

Other Gloucestershire material is noted in:

HOWES, R. 'The Historical Manuscripts Commission and local history', *Local history bulletin* **47**, 1983, 2-5.

3. JOURNALS AND NEWSPAPERS

Every genealogist with ancestors from Gloucestershire or Bristol should subscribe to at least one of the family history society journals for the county:
Journal of the Gloucestershire Family History Society [ ]: the Society, 1979- . This is indexed in: GLOUCESTERSHIRE FAMILY HISTORY SOCIETY. *Index to journals* **1-12**. [ ]: the Society, *c*.1982. Further separate indexes covering vols. **13-24** and **25-36** were issued *c*.1985 and in 1989 respectively.
Journal of the Bristol & Avon Family History Society. Bristol: the Society, 1975- . This is indexed in: KENT, BARBARA, 'Quinquennial index of the Bristol & Avon Family History Society, journals **1-20**, 1975-80', *J.B.A.* **21**, 1980, ixv.
By stream and staple: the journal of the Wotton under Edge Family History Group. Wotton: the Group 1989- .

The most important general historical journal, which contains much information of genealogical value, is:
Bristol & Gloucestershire Archaeological Society transactions. Bristol: the Society, 1876- . This is indexed in: JONES, WILLIAM. *General index to volumes I-XX, 1876-1897*. Gloucester: H. Osborne, 1900. AUSTIN, ROLAND. *General index to volumes XXI-XL, covering the years 1898-1917, with a subject index to the illustrations in volumes I-XL*. Gloucester: J.W. Arrowsmith for the Society, 1919. AUSTIN, ROLAND, *General index to volumes 41-50, 1918-1929 ...* Gloucester: the Society, 1930. AUSTIN, ROLAND, *General index to volumes 51-60 (1930-1939) ...* Gloucester: H. Osborne for the Society, 1942. RICHARDSON, EILEEN M., *General index to volumes 61-70 (1939-1951)*. Gloucester: John Bellows for the Society, 1956. RICHARDSON, EILEEN M., *General index to volumes 71-78 (1952-1959)*. Gloucester: John Bellows for the Society, 1962. MORGAN, KATHLEEN, *General index to volumes 79-90 (1960-1971)*. Gloucester: the Society, 1974, and VAUGHAN, SUSAN, *General index to volumes 91-100 (1972-1982)*. [Gloucester]: [the Society], [1984?].
Of even greater value to the genealogist is:
Gloucestershire notes & queries. 10 vols. Bristol: W George *et al.*, 1881-1914. Discontinued 1905, resumed 1913-1914, and indexed in: RICHARDSON, EILEEN M., *Gloucestershire notes & queries: general index*. Gloucester: Gloucestershire Community Council, (Local History Committee), 1956.

The publications of record societies often include works vital to the genealogist. Many are listed in the following chapters. The two major series for the county are:
Bristol & Gloucestershire Archaeological Society Records Branch. Bristol: the Society, 1952- .
Bristol Record Society publications. Bristol: the Society, 1930- .
Other county-wide journals include:
Gloucestershire local history newsletter. Gloucester: Gloucestershire Community Council, 1979- . Mainly society news and announcements, with listing of new publications etc.
Gloucestershire historical studies: studies in local historical records by the University Extra-Mural class at Gloucester. Bristol: University of Bristol Dept. of Extra-Mural Studies, 1966-1980.
Local history bulletin. 54 vols. Whaddon: Gloucestershire Community Council, 1952-86. Continued by: *Gloucestershire history*. Gloucester: Gloucestershire Rural Community Council, 1987- . Includes much information on local history, mainly brief notes.
A number of useful local journals are also available:
Avon past. Avon Archaeological Council/Avon Local History Association, 1979- .
Charlton Kings Local History Society bulletin. Charlton Kings: the Society, 1979- . A detailed name index is provided in: *Charlton Kings Local History Society research bulletin indexes: volumes 1-7 (Spring 1979 - Spring 1982)*. Charlton Kings, the Society, 1985.
Cheltenham Local History Society journal. Cheltenham: the Society, 1983- .
Clifton Antiquarian Club proceedings. Bristol: the Club, 1884-1912. There is an index to vols **1-7**, 1884-1912, in **7**, 219-41.
Cotteswold Naturalists Field Club proceedings. London: the Club, 1847-53. This is indexed in: AUSTIN, ROLAND, *Index to the Proceedings of the Cotteswold Naturalists Field Club, volumes I-XVII, 1846-1912*. London: J. Wheldon & Co., 1913.
History of Tetbury Society journal. Tetbury: the Society, 1984- .
For newspapers, see:
BRISTOL PUBLIC LIBRARIES. *Early Bristol newspapers: a detailed catalogue of Bristol newspapers published up to and including the year 1800 in the Bristol Reference Library*. Bristol: Corporation of Bristol, 1956.

Journals and Newspapers continued

MYLES-HOOK, C. 'Bristol newspapers', *J.B.A.* **51**, 1988, 33-37. List of 18-19th c. newspapers at Bristol Central Library.

4. NAMES AND DIALECT

Where is Wheatenhurst? Obscure place names are constantly cropping up in genealogical research. To identify them, consult:
SMITH, A.H., ed. *The place names of Gloucestershire*. English Place Name Society, **38-41**. Cambridge: Cambridge University Press, 1964-65.
See also:
BADDELEY, W.St.C. *Place names of Gloucestershire: a handbook*. Gloucester: John Bellows, 1913.
Bristol place name changes are listed in:
'Place name changes', *J.B.A.* **32**, 1983, 8-10, and **33**, 1983, 10-12. In Bristol.
For Bristol topography, consult:
Arrowsmith's dictionary of Bristol. 2nd ed. Bristol: J.W. Arrowsmith, 1906.
The study of personal names may also be of interest to genealogists. Two recent essays in this field are:
FRANKLIN, PETER. 'Normans, saints and politics: forename choice among fourteenth-century Gloucestershire peasants', *Local population studies* **36**, 1986, 19-26. Study of name giving in Thornbury.
PENN, SIMON. 'The origins of Bristol migrants in the early fourteenth century: the surname evidence', *B.G.A.S.Tr.* **101**, 1983, 123-30.
Dialect words may also cause you problems. To solve them, a number of dialect glossaries are available:
HUNTLEY, RICHARD WEBSTER. *A glossary of the Cotswold (Gloucestershire) dialect*. J.R. Smith, 1868.
LEMMON, C.H. 'The native speech of Gloucestershire', *B.G.A.S.Tr.* **64**, 1943, 164-210. Includes extensive glossary.
ROBERTSON, J. DRUMMOND. *A glossary of dialect and archaic words used in the county of Gloucester*, ed. Lord Moreton. English Dialect Society publications **61**, series **C**. Kegan Paul, Trench, Trubner & Co, 1890.
A glossary of provincial words used in Gloucestershire with proverbs current in that country. John Gray Bell, 1851.
LAWSON, ROBERT. *Upton on Severn words and phrases*. English Dialect Society, 1884.

5. BIOGRAPHICAL DICTIONARIES, GENEALOGICAL DIRECTORIES AND OCCUPATIONAL LISTS

Amongst the most valuable sources of genealogical information are the directories of members' interests published by the various family history societies. These provide the names and addresses of their members, together with a list of surnames being researched. If yours is listed, maybe much of the work has been done! Or at least, someone may be willing to share the work. See:
GLOUCESTERSHIRE FAMILY HISTORY SOCIETY. *Directory of names in which members are interested*. 4th ed. [ ]: G.F.H.S., 1988.
BRISTOL & AVON FAMILY HISTORY SOCIETY. *Directory of members interests*. Bristol: the Society, 1991. To be updated annually.

Biographical dictionaries provide brief biographical information on the individuals listed. Many such dictionaries are available, and are invaluable to the genealogist. For general guidance on identifying them, consult *English genealogy: an introductory bibliography*. Many are listed in *Occupational sources for genealogists*.

Gloucestershire:
GASKELL, ERNEST. *Gloucestershire leaders: social and political*. Queenhithe Printing, 1906.
STACEY, C. *Men of the West: a pictorial who's who of the distinguished, eminent and famous men of the West Country, embracing the counties of Cornwall, Devon, Somerset, Dorset, Wilts and Gloucester, including the city of Bristol*. Claude Stacey Limited, 1926.
STRATFORD, JOSEPH. *Good and great men of Gloucester: A series of biographical sketches, with a brief history of the county*. Cirencester: C.H. Savoy, 1867. This is continued by:
STRATFORD, JOSEPH. *Gloucester biographical notes*. Gloucester: The Journal Office, 1887. Includes 35 biographical sketches originally published in the *Gloucester Journal*.
'Dictionary of national biography: list of Gloucestershire biographical sketches', *G.N.Q.* **4**, 1890, 614-9. List of Gloucestershire entries in the *Dictionary of national biography*. Covers vols. **1-10**, A-Clark, only; not continued.
Gloucestershire lives: social and political. Truman Press, [1894].
Who's Who in Gloucestershire. Hereford: Wilson & Phillips, 1934.

Biographical Dictionaries etc. continued

Bristol
FREEMAN, A.B. *Bristol worthies and notable residents in the district, past and present.* Bristol: Burleigh, 1907. 2nd series issued 1909.

PRYCE, GEORGE. *A popular history of Bristol, antiquarian, topographical, and descriptive, from the earliest period to the present time, with biographical notices of eminent natives.* Bristol: W. Mack, 1861. Includes biographical notices of leading inhabitants.

Cheltenham
Who's Who in Cheltenham. Newport: William Press, [1910].

Forest of Dean
NICHOLLS, H.G. *The personalities of the Forest of Dean, being a relation of its successive officials, gentry, and commonalty.* J. Murray, 1863

Gloucester
Who's Who in Gloucester. Newport on Usk: Williams Press, 1910.

For Freemasons, see:
NORMAN, GEORGE. *Freemasonry: Provincial Grand Lodge of Gloucestershire, with some account of the older lodges of the Province.* Cheltenham: the author, 1911. Includes lists of officers, etc.
POWELL, ARTHUR CECIL, & LITTLETON, JOSEPH. *A history of freemasonry in Bristol.* Bristol: Berrett Bros., 1910. Includes lists of officers *etc.*
The Freemasons' calendar and directory for the Province of Gloucester. Gloucester: John Bellows, 1879-1965. Annual; includes list of members.

There are many works offering biographical information on persons of particular occupations. These are listed here. For clergymen, see chapter 13, for members of parliament and local government officers, chapter 15, for teachers and students, chapter 16.

Apprentices
Bristol apprentices are listed in:
Calendar of the Bristol apprentice book, 1532-1565. Bristol Record Society publications, **14**, **33**, and ?, Bristol: the Society, 1949- . Contents: 1. 1532-1542, ed. D. Hollis. 2. 1542-1552, ed. Elizabeth Ralph & Nora M. Hardwick. 3. Not yet issued.

Apprentices *continued*

McGREGOR, MARGARET, ed. *Bristol apprentices book. 1566-1573.* Bristol: Bristol & Avon Family History Society, [198-]. List of apprentices, continued by: McGREGOR, MARGARET, ed. *Bristol apprentice book, 1573-1578.* Bristol: Bristol & Avon Family History Society, 1990.

GOODMAN, W.L. 'Bristol apprentice register 1532-1658: a selection of enrolments of mariners', *Mariners mirror* **60**, 1974, 27-31. Includes names.

GOODMAN, W.L. 'Musical instruments and their makers in Bristol apprentice registers, 1536-1643', *Galpin Society Journal* **28**, 1974, 9-14. Includes extracts from the registers.

JONES, I. FITZROY. 'Apprenticeship books of Bristol', *Genealogists' magazine* **8**(1), 1938, 10-13. [1532-1849]. Brief note only.

YARBROUGH, ANNE. 'Geographical and social origins of Bristol apprentices, 1542-1565', *B.G.A.S.Tr.* **98**, 1980, 113-29. No names, but obvious implications for genealogists.

WILLIAMS, JOHN. 'Bristol apprentice books', *J.B.A.* **52**, 1988, 25-5. Brief discussion of books running from 1532 to the present day.

For apprentices in other places, see:
GREET, M.J. 'Apprenticeships and bastardy: a review of the Charlton records', *C.K.L.H.S.B.* **9**, 1983, 34-6. Includes list of names with biographical notes.

MARSH, BOWER. 'Apprentices from the county of Gloucester bound at Carpenters Hall, London, 1654-1694', *G.N.Q.* **10**, 1914, 76-80. Not continued.

Architects
GOMME, ANDOR, JENNER, MICHAEL, & LITTLE, BRIAN. *Bristol: an architectural history.* Lund Humphries, 1979. Includes biographical dictionary of Bristol architects.

Bell-founders
WALTERS, H.B. 'The Gloucestershire bell-foundries', *B.G.A.S.Tr.* **34**, 1911, 110-19.

Boatmen
'1851 census: waterways', *J.G.F.H.S.* **8**, 1981, 24-6; **10**, 1981, 9-11; **13**, 1982, 15-16. Gloucestershire boatmen in Worcestershire.

Builders
POWELL, CHRISTOPHER. 'Widows and others on Bristol building sites: some women in nineteenth century construction', *Local historian* **20**, 1990, 84-7. Includes brief lists of builders.

Biographical Dictionaries etc. continued

Clockmakers
BUCKLEY, FRANCIS, & BUCKLEY, GEORGE B. 'Clock and watch makers of the 18th century in Gloucestershire and Bristol, compiled from directories, poll-books, and newspapers', *B.G.A.S.Tr.* **51**, 1929, 305-19.

DOWLER, GRAHAM. *Gloucestershire clock and watchmakers.* Chichester: Phillimore, 1984. Includes directory of makers, with ten pedigrees, and biographical notes.

NOTT, H.E. & HUDLESTON, C. ROY. 'An 18th century clock at the Council House, Bristol, with notes on clock and watchmakers in Bristol', *B.G.A.S.Tr.* **57**, 1935, 176-91. Alphabetical list. See also Goldsmiths.

Clothiers
CLUTTERBUCK, R.H. 'State papers relating to the cloth trade, 1622', *B.G.A.S.Tr.* **5**, 1880-1, 154-62. Includes list of Gloucestershire clothiers, 1621.

Convicts
BROAD, IAN R. 'Bristol executions', *J.B.A.* **53**, 1988, 37-9. List, 18-19th c.

DEVERILL, PENNY. 'Lawford's Gate Prison, Bristol', *J.B.A.* **61**, 1990, 30-31. List of prisoners, 1820.

PHILLIPS, JUDITH. 'Bristol executions, 1741-1841', *J.B.A.* **1**, 1875, 33-4. Includes list. See also page 75.

Cordwainers
ELRINGTON, C.R. 'Records of the Cordwainers' Society of Tewkesbury, 1562-1941', *B.G.A.S.Tr.* **85**, 1966, 164-174. Includes description of the Society's archives.

Glass-makers
BUCKLEY, FRANCIS. 'The early glasshouses of Bristol', *Transactions of the Society of Glass Technology* **9**, 1925, 36-61. Includes names of glass-makers.

POWELL, ARTHUR CECIL. 'Glass-making in Bristol', *B.G.A.S.Tr.* **47**, 1925, 211-57. Includes notes on many glass-makers.

Goldsmiths
MORTON, H.E., & HUDLESTON, C. ROY. 'Bristol gold and silversmiths and clock and watchmakers', *B.G.A.S.Tr.* **60**, 1938, 198-227. Alphabetical list.

Highwaymen
LINDEGAARD, PATRICIA. 'Highwaymen of Bristol', *J.B.A.* **36**, 1984, 17-19.

Horse-dealers
LEWIN, RON. '18th century horse dealers in Bristol', *J.B.A.* **45**, 1986, 32-4. Lists names and parishes of buyers and sellers.

Librarians
EWARD, SUZANNE MARY. *A catalogue of Gloucester Cathedral Library.* Gloucester: Dean and Chapter, 1972. Includes list of librarians from 1660, but not much else of genealogical interest.

Licensees
A list of licensed houses in the Campden petty session division, with names of occupiers, lessees, owners, &c., &c. Gloucester: Offices of the Clerk of the Standing Joint Committee for Gloucestershire, 1891.

A list of all licensed houses in the county of Gloucestershire, with names of occupiers, lessees, owners, hours of closing &c. Gloucester: Court of Quarter Sessions, 1903. See also victuallers.

Merchants
EBERLE, E.F. 'List of the Merchants Hall, Bristol, 1732', *B.G.A.S.Tr.* **11**, 1886-7, 291-2.

LATIMER, JOHN. *History of the Society of Merchant Venturers of the City of Bristol, with some account of the anterior merchants' guilds.* Bristol: J.W. Arrowsmith, 1903. Includes lists of masters, wardens and treasurers, 1500-1902.

McGRATH, PATRICK, ed. *Merchants and merchandise in seventeenth century Bristol.* Bristol Record Society publications **19**. Bristol: the Society, 1955. Includes many wills and probate inventories.

McGRATH, PATRICK. *The Merchant Venturers of Bristol: a history of the Society of Merchant Venturers of the City of Bristol from its origin to the present day.* Bristol: the Society, 1975. Includes register of members, 1800-1974 *etc.*

McGRATH, PATRICK, ed. *Records relating to the Society of Merchant Venturers of the City of Bristol in the seventeenth century.* Bristol Record Society publications **17**. Bristol: the Society, 1952. Includes names of many merchants, ship owners *etc.*

MINCHINTON, W.E., ed. *The trade of Bristol in the eighteenth century.* Bristol Record Society publications **20**. Bristol: the Society, 1957. Includes names of many merchants, ship owners *etc.*

RICHARDSON, DAVID. *Bristol, Africa, and the eighteenth century slave trade to America.* Bristol Record Society publications **38-9**. Bristol: the Society, 1986-7. Lists vessels and owners. See also Seamen.

Biographical Dictionaries etc. continued

Millers
MILLS, STEPHEN & RIEMER, PIERCE. *The mills of Gloucestershire*. Buckingham: Barracuda Books, 1989. Gives names of many millers in the course of tracing the history of mills.

Miners
LINDEGAARD, PATRICIA. 'The colliers' trade: a Bristol incident of 1753', *J.B.A.* **11**, 1978, 8-10. Includes list of Kingswood colliery rioters.
LINDEGAARD, PATRICIA. 'Killed in a coalpit', *J.B.A.* **19**, 1980, 21-4. Death extracts from parish registers and local newspapers, 18-19th c.
LINDEGAARD, PATRICIA. *Killed in a coalpit*. 3 vols. (projected). Kingswood: V. Britton, c.1988- . List of fatalities, 1700-1930, with brief biographical notices.
LINDEGAARD, PATRICIA. 'South Gloucestershire colliery children and young people', *J.B.A.* **12**, 1978, 28-9. List from a parliamentary paper of 1841.
LINDEGAARD, PATRICIA. 'The underground men (a colliers' index)', *J.G.F.H.S.* **7**, 1980, 12-13. Lists surnames frequently appearing in the author's ms. index. See also **8**, 1981, 10, and *J.B.A.* **24**, 1981, 14-15.

Pewterers
COTTERELL, HOWARD HERSCHELL. *Bristol and West Country pewterers, with illustrations of their marks*. Bristol: A.W. Ford & Co., 1918. Includes list with brief biographical notes.

Physicians
B[LACKER], B.H. 'Munk's roll of physicians: Gloucestershire names', *G.N.Q.* **4**, 1890, 486-93.

Pipemakers
PRICE, ROGER, JACKSON, REG. & JACKSON, PHILOMENA. *Bristol clay pipe makers*. Rev. ed. Bristol: the authors, 1979. List with many biographical details.

Police
JERRARD, BRYAN. 'Police history in Gloucestershire and family history', *J.G.F.H.S.* **13**, 1982, 5-7 Useful discussion of sources.

Potters
JACKSON, REG. & PHILOMENA, & PRICE, ROGER. *Bristol potters and potteries*. Journal of ceramic history **12**. Stoke: Stoke on Trent City Museum, 1982. List with much biographical information.

Potters continued

POUNTNEY, W.J. *Old Bristol potteries, being an account of the old potters and potteries of Bristol and Brislington, between 1650 and 1850, with some pages on the old Chapel of St Anne, Brislington*. Bristol: J.W.A. Arrowsmith, 1920. Includes extensive list of Bristol apprentices, and of potters in the burgess rolls.

Printers
HYETT, F.A. 'Notes on the first Bristol and Gloucestershire printers', *B.G.A.S.Tr.* **20**, 1895-96, 38-51.

Ropemakers
WEBB, FRED. G. Bristol and the rope trade', *Notes on Bristol history* **5**, 1962, 41-51. Includes list of 18-19th c. ropemakers.

Seamen
AUSTIN, BARBARA. 'Bristol shipping records', *J.B.A.* **49**, 1987, 25.
FARR, GRAHAM E., ed. *Records of Bristol ships, 1800-1838 (vessels over 150 tons)*, Bristol Record Society publications **15**. Bristol: the Society, 1950. Includes names of owners and masters.
MINCHINTON, W.E., ed. *Politics and the port of Bristol in the eighteenth century: the petitions of the Society of Merchant Venturers, 1698-1803*. Bristol Record Society publications **23**. Bristol: the Society, 1963. Includes register of members, lists of Bristol pilots, haven masters and ballast masters *etc.*
ROE, MICHAEL, ed. *The journal and letters of Captain Charles Bishop on the north west coast of America, in the Pacific, and in New South Wales, 1794-1799*. Hakluyt Society, 2nd series, **131**. The Society, 1967. Includes crew lists of Bristol ships.
POWELL, J.W. DAMER. 'Lists of Bristol ships, 1571 and 1572', *B.G.A.S.Tr.* **52**, 1930, 117-22. Includes names of masters.
POWELL, J.W. DAMER 'Somerset ships', *Notes & queries for Somerset & Dorset* **20**, 1930-2, 124-7. Includes names of mariners of Bristol and Somerset, 1570.
'Port of Burnham on Sea: 1881 census', *J.G.F.H.S.* **27**, 1985, 9-10. Gloucestershire mariners.
See also Apprentices and Merchants.

Shipbuilders
FARR, GRAHAME. *Shipbuilding in the Port of Bristol*. Maritime monographs and reports **27**. Greenwich: National Maritime Museum, 1977. Includes notes on many 18-19th c. shipbuilders.

Biographical Dictionaries etc. continued

Ship Owners
See Merchants and seamen.

Soapmakers
MATTHEWS, HAROLD EVAN, ed. *Proceedings, minutes, and enrolments of the company of soapmakers, 1562-1642.* Bristol Record Society publications **10**. Bristol: the Society, 1940.

Soldiers and Militiamen *etc.*
Many men of Gloucestershire and Bristol served in the Army, or in the militia, and much information on them is available in the various regimental histories *etc.* which have have been compiled. These cannot all be listed here. The works included below include only those publications which provide lists of officers and men, and which are therefore of direct interest to the genealogist. The list is in chronological order.

O'FLYNN, G. 'Gloucestershire trained bands', *Notes & queries* **167**, 1934, 93-5 and 111-13. List of some members, 1608.

BRODIGAN, F., ed. *Historical records of the twenty-eighth North Gloucestershire Regiment, from 1692 to 1882.* Blackfriars, 1884. Includes various lists of officers *etc.*

'Payments relating to militia services, 1780-1814', *C.K.L.H.S.B.* **2**, 1979, 14-20. Includes list of Charlton Kings men appointing substitutes.

'Deserters from the South Battalion, Gloucestershire militia', *J.G.F.H.S.* **39**, 1988, 22. List, 1791.

BULLOCK, H. 'Gloucestershire volunteers, 1795-1815: an alphabetical list of artillery and infantry volunteer corps in Gloucester', *Journal of the Society for Army Historical Research* **38**, 1960, 76-82. List of the various corps, with names of commanding officers.

AUSTIN, ROLAND. 'The early years of the Royal Gloucester Yeomanry Cavalry', *B.G.A.S.Tr.* **43**, 1921, 253-66. Includes list of officers, 1797-1823, with other names.

'Gloucestershire militia men in 1797', *B.G.A.S.Tr.* **64**, 1943, 148-57. List of men from the hundreds of Britwells Barrow and Bradley.

BROWN, JAMES. *The rise, progress, and military improvement of the Bristol volunteers, with an alphabetical list of the officers and privates.* Bristol: W. Matthews, 1798. Reprinted Bristol: Bristol Times & Mirror, 1916.

'The Longtree, Bisley and Whitstone Volunteer Cavalry', *G.N.Q.* **1**, 1881, 424-7. Roll of members, 1798.

Soldiers and Militiamen continued

MICHELL, G.B., 'Frampton volunteers, 1798-1802', *Journal of the Society for Army Historical Research* **7**, 1928, 219-21. Includes names of officers.

'Gloucestershire militia, 1803', *J.G.F.H.S.* **37**, 1988, 15-16. List of names, with abodes.

WILKINS, H.J. *History of the Loyal Westbury Volunteer Corps from A.D. 1803 to A.D. 1814.* Bristol: J.W. Arrowsmith, 1918. Includes list of volunteers, with ages and marital status and many other names.

WILLIAMS, J. ROBERT. 'Gloucestershire pensioners of the 43rd foot', *J.G.F.H.S.* **28**, 1986, 6-9. List of those who became Chelsea Pensioners, 1806-38.

WILLIAMS, J.R. 'The blind half hundred', *J.G.F.H.S.* **21**, 1984, 6-12. Includes list of Gloucestershire men in the 50th Foot, 1809-27.

CRIPPS, WILFRED JOSEPH. *The Royal North Gloucestershire Militia.* [Reprinted with additions]. Cirencester: Wilts. & Gloucestershire Standard Printing Works, [1915]. Includes roll of officers, 1852-1908, and other names from 1780.

'Details from a memorial to be seen in Cheltenham', *J.G.F.H.S.* **10**, 1981, 15-16. To those who fell in the Crimea.

Annual list of the Bristol and Gloucestershire Artillery Corps. Bristol: Rose & Harris, 1867. Full list of members.

War in South Africa: some Gloucestershire officers and volunteers at the front: a local souvenir. Gloucester: Gloucester Journal, 1899-1900. 27 portraits, with short biographical notes.

FOX, FRANK. *The history of the Royal Gloucestershire Hussars Yeomanry 1898-1922: the great cavalry campaign in Palestine.* Philip Allan, 1923. Includes roll of honour, and list of subscribers to war memorial, with many other names.

Soldiers died in the Great War, 1914-19. Part 33: The Gloucestershire Regiment. H.M.S.O., 1921. Reprinted Polstead: J.B. Hayward & Son, 1988.

BARNES, A.F. ed. *The story of the 2/5th battalion Gloucestershire Regiment 1914-1918.* Gloucester: Crypt House Press, 1930. Includes list of fatalities, noting cemetery or memorial, and lists of those who gained distinctions.

PITMAN, STUART. *Second Royal Gloucestershire Hussars: Libya, Egypt 1941-1942.* Saint Catherine Press, 1950. Includes rolls of honour.

Biographical Dictionaries etc. continued

Soldiers and Militiamen *continued*

CAREW, TIM. *The glorious Glosters.* Leo Cooper, 1970. Covers 1945-70, and includes list of honours and awards.

Tradesmen

In an age when coins were in short supply, a variety of tradesmen issued their own tokens. Studies of these tokens often provides information of genealogical value. See:

BRAVENDER, T.B. 'List of tokens found at Cirencester', *B.G.A.S.Tr.* **8**, 1883-4, 314-23.

D., C.T. 'Some Gloucestershire tokens of the seventeenth century', *G.N.Q.* **3**, 1887, 284-6.

GRAY, IRVINE. 'Some seventeenth century token-issuers', *B.G.A.S.Tr.* **84**, 1965, 101-9. General discussion, with some names.

PRITCHARD, JOHN E. 'Bristol tokens of the sixteenth and seventeenth centuries, with special reference to the square farthings', *Proceedings of the Clifton Antiquarian Club* **4**, 1897-99, 277-89. Includes brief list of tokens issued by private traders.

WILTON, JOHN PLEYDELL. 'Gloucester tokens of the 17th, 18th and 19th centuries', *B.G.A.S.Tr.* **13**, 1888-9, 130-45.

'Numismata Glocestriensia'. 1650-70. *G.N.Q.* **1**, 1881, 347-52. List of traders' tokens.

Victuallers

'Gloucestershire victuallers, 1755: Glocester: Hundred of Berkeley Upper', *J.G.F.H.S.* **36**, 1988, 29-30 and **37**, 1988, 17-18. List of 80 victuallers, with names of their inns and sureties. See also Licensees.

Watchmakers

See Clockmakers.

Weavers

LEWIN, RON. 'Bristol weavers in 1738', *J.B.A.* **60**, 1990. List of weavers presented to the Princess of Wales.

6. VISITATION RETURNS AND HERALDRY

In the sixteenth and seventeenth centuries, the heralds undertook 'visitations' of the counties in order to determine the rights of gentry to bear heraldic arms. One consequence of this activity was the compilation of pedigrees of most of the gentry. The heralds' returns continue to be important sources of genealogical information; for Gloucestershire, see:

BANNERMAN, W. BRUCE, ed. 'The visitation of Glocestershire', *M.G.H.*, 4th series, **5**, 1912-13, 157-66, 205-13, 237-43, 285-92 and 333-9. Apparently from the visitation of 1582-3.

MACLEAN, SIR JOHN, & HEANE, W.C., eds. *The visitation of the county of Gloucester, taken in the year 1623 by Henry Chitty and John Phillipot as deputies to William Camden, Clarenceaux King of Arms, with pedigrees from the Heralds' visitations of 1569 and 1582-3, and sundry miscellaneous pedigrees.* Harleian Society visitations **21**. The Society, 1885.

FENWICK, T. FITZROY, & METCALFE, WALTER C., eds. *The visitation of the county of Gloucester begun by Thomas May, Chester, and Gregory King, Rouge Dragon, and finished by Henry Dethick, Richmond, and the said Rouge Dragon, Pursuivant, in Trinity Vacacon, 1683, by virtue of several deputacons from Sir Henry St. George, Clarenceaux King of Arms.* Exeter: William Pollard, 1884.

CONDER, EDWARD. 'Some notes on the visitations of Gloucestershire', *B.G.A.S.Tr.* **28**, 1905, 124-30. Includes list of Gloucestershire material at the College of Arms.

For heraldry, see:

A collection of coats of arms borne by the nobility and gentry of the county of Glocester. J Good, 1792.

SUMMERS, PETER. ed. *Hatchments in Britain* **7**: *Cornwall, Devon, Dorset, Gloucestershire, Hampshire, Isle of Wight and Somerset.* Phillimore, 1988.

WERE, F. 'Index to the heraldry in Bigland's *History of Gloucestershire* with notes', *B.G.A.S.Tr.* **28**, 1905, 147-509.

WERE, F. 'Notes on the heraldry on the maps in T. Chubb's *Descriptive catalogue of the printed maps of Gloucestershire*' *B.G.A.S.Tr.* **37**, 1914, 235-9.

Visitation Returns and Heraldry continued

Were also gave a number of papers on local heraldry at meetings of the Bristol & Gloucestershire Archaeological Society. One or two other papers of use are also noted here:

Bath:
WERE, F. 'Heraldry as read ... during the ... Society's meeting at Bath', *B.G.A.S.Tr.* **23**, 1900, 99-128. See **28**, 1905, 510, for correction. Despite being read in Bath, does include notes on Gloucestershire heraldry.

Berkeley
WERE, F., 'Heraldic notes of the spring excursion to Berkeley Castle', *B.G.A.S.Tr.* **28**, 1905, 86-8.

Bristol
CONDER, EDWARD & WERE, FRANCIS. 'The heraldry of some of the citizens of Bristol between 1662 and 1688', *B.G.A.S.Tr.* **30**, 1907, 273-82.
WERE, F. 'Bristol Cathedral heraldry', *B.G.A.S.Tr.* **25**, 1902, 102-32.
WERE, F. 'Heraldry in Red Lodge, Bristol', *B.G.A.S.Tr.* **24**, 1901, 262-6.
WOODWARD, JOHN. 'The heraldry of Bristol Cathedral', *Herald & genealogist* **4**, 1867, 289-309.

Cheltenham
WERE, F. 'Notes on heraldry in churches during Cheltenham meeting', *B.G.A.S.Tr.* **28**, 1905, 89-93.

Chipping Camden
WERE, F. 'Heraldry: read ... during Chipping Camden meeting', *B.G.A.S.Tr.* **25**, 1902, 187-211.

Dymock
WERE, F. 'A few notes on the heraldry seen at the spring meeting, June 2nd, 1908', *B.G.A.S.Tr.* **31**, 1908, 284-7. At Dymock, Kempley and Pauntley.

Fairford
WERE, F. 'Heraldry of the different churches, &c., visited by the Gloucestershire Archaeological Society during their visit to Fairford, August 9th to 11th, 1899', *B.G.A.S.Tr.* **22**, 1899, 138-49.

Kempley
See Dymock.

Pauntley
See Dymock.

Tewkesbury
WERE, F. 'Heraldry in Tewkesbury Abbey', *B.G.A.S.Tr.* **26**(1), 1903, 162-72.

Toddington
WERE, F. 'Heraldic notes made ... during the excursion to Toddington on June 7th, 1900', *B.G.A.S.Tr.* **23**, 1900, 96-8. Mainly from Stanton Church and Stanway House.

Winterbourne
WERE, F. 'Heraldry: Winterbourne Church', *B.G.A.S.Tr.* **25**, 1902, 183-7.

7. FAMILY HISTORIES

Adeane
See Dene

Agg
'Hewletts and the Agg family', *Cheltenham Local History Society Journal*, **5**, 1987, 11-22. 19th c.

Alye
'The family of Alye', *Herald & genealogist* **6**, 1871, 223-31. Of Tewkesbury, includes pedigrees, 17th c.

Annesley
'Royal and baronial descents of the families of Annesley, Cotton, Booth, Tyndale, and others', *B.G.A.S.Tr.* **14**, 1889-90, 101-16.

Apsley
HANKEY, JULIA ALEXANDER. *History of the Apsley and Bathurst families.* Cirencester: E.W. Savory, 1889. Includes pedigree, 14-17th c. Another edition, compiled by A.B. Bathurst, was published Cirencester: G.H. Harmer, 1903.

Archard
LINDLEY, E.S. 'William Archard: an unrecognised Gloucestershire worthy', *B.G.A.S.Tr.* **68**, 1949, 190-7. Includes pedigree, 16-17th c.

Arrowsmith
FLETCHER, W.G. DINNOCK. 'The family of Arrowsmith', *G.N.Q.* **5**, 1894, 432-7. 17-18th c. pedigree.

Arundell
ARUNDELL, EDWARD. 'The Arundells of Gloucestershire,' *B.G.A.S.Tr.* **66**, 1947, 208-18. 15-16th c.

Astry
See Chester.

Atkyns
AUSTIN, ROLAND. Some account of Sir Robert Atkyns the Younger and other members of the Atkyns family', *B.G.A.S.Tr.* **35**, 1912, 69-92. 17-18th c.

Avenel
MACLEAN, SIR JOHN. 'Family of Avenel', *B.G.A.S.Tr.* **4**, 1879-80, 313-9. Includes pedigree, 12-14th c.

Barclay
BARCLAY, CHARLES W., et al. *History of the Barclay family with full pedigree from 1066 to [1933].* 3 vols. St. Catherine Press, 1924-34. Contents: 1 [Gloucestershire family, by Charles W. Barclay.]. **2**. The Barclays in Scotland from 1067 to 1660, by Hubert F. Barclay. **3**. The Barclays in Scotland and England, by Hubert F. Barclay & Alice Wilson-Fox. Apart from Gloucestershire and Scotland, the family also had branches in London (where a member founded Barclays Bank); Walthamstow, Essex; and Bury Hill, Dorking, Surrey.
See also Berkeley.

Barnard
ONIONS, K. 'A poor family from Mitcheldean', in SMITH, B.S., ed. *Studies in Dean history.* Bristol: University of Bristol Dept. of Extra-Mural Studies, 1963. Barnard family, late 18th c. Includes pedigree.

Barnes
BARNES, ARTHUR HARMAN. *History of a family: Barnes.* Ormskirk: [the author?], 1967-8. Of Frome, Somerset, Bristol, Herefordshire, and Reading, Berkshire. Includes pedigree, 17-20th c.

Barrow
CRAWLEY-BOEVEY, ARTHUR WILLIAM. 'Pedigree of Sir Charles Barrow, Bart., of Highgrove, Minsterworth, co. Gloucester', *Genealogist*, N.S. **30**, 1914, 73-86.
See also Paulet.

Bartlett
BOWEN, ELIZABETH. 'The Bartlett family, Bristol wine merchants', *J.B.A.* **18**, 1979, 7-10. See also **19**, 1980, 31.

Bathurst
'The Bathurst family of Lechlade', *G.N.Q.* **1**, 1881, 369-71.
See also Apsley.

Batten
PAGET, M. 'The Knappings, and its occupiers', *C.K.L.H.S.B.* **23**, 1990, 20-25. Includes pedigrees of Batten, 17-18th c., and Currier, 16-17th c.

Berkeley
BARKLY, SIR HENRY. 'The Berkeleys of Cobberley', *B.G.A.S.Tr.* **17**, 1892-3, 96-125. 12-15th c.
BARKLY, SIR HENRY. 'The Berkeleys of Dursley', *B.G.A.S.Tr.* **13**, 1888-9, 188-95.

Family Histories continued

Berkeley continued

BARKLY, SIR HENRY. 'The Berkeleys of Dursley during the 13th and 14th centuries', *B.G.A.S.Tr.* **9**, 1884-5, 227-76. Includes pedigree, and list of tenants of Dodington sued in 1287.

BARKLY, SIR HENRY. 'The earlier house of Berkeley', *B.G.A.S.Tr.* **8**, 1883-4, 193-223. Includes pedigree, 11-13th c.

BARKLY, SIR HENRY. 'The earliest pipe roll', *Genealogist*, N.S. **3**, 1886, 79. Berkeley family, 11th c.

BARRON, OSWALD. 'Our oldest families, X: the Berkeleys', *Ancestor* **8**, Jan 1904, 73-81. 11-19th c.

CLAY, SIR CHARLES. 'The marriages of Robert, son of Robert, son of Harding', *B.G.A.S.Tr.* **80**, 1961, 90-92. Berkeley forebears, medieval.

COOKE, JAMES HERBERT. 'The Berkeley manuscripts and their author, John Smyth', *B.G.A.S.Tr.* **5**, 1880-1, 212-21. Notes on Smyth's works, then in mss, i.e., *Lives of the Berkeleys, Description of the Hundred of Berkeley*, list of freeholders of Berkeley Hundred *etc*.

FINBERG, H.P.R. 'Three studies in family history', in his *Gloucestershire studies*. Leicester: Leicester University Press, 1957, 145-83. Berkeley of Berkeley, Kingscote of Kingscote, and Holder of Taynton.

FOSBROOKE, THOMAS DUDLEY. *Berkeley manuscripts: abstracts and extracts of Smyth's lives of the Berkeleys ... including all the pedigrees in the ancient manuscript, to which are annexed a copious history of the castle and parish of Berkeley ... and biographical anecdotes of Dr Jenner*. J. Nichols & Son, 1821.

KENNEDY-SKIPTON, H.S. 'The Berkeleys at Yate', *B.G.A.S.Tr.* **21**, 1898, 25-31. 15-17th c.

LINDLEY, E.S. 'Some early Berkeley ladies', *B.G.A.S.Tr.* **84**, 1965, 31-43. Medieval.

MOORE, MATTEY. 'Berkeley Castle yesterday and today', *Connoisseur* **137**, 1956, 241-8. Berkeley family, brief summary.

SINCLAIR, ALEXANDRA. 'The great Berkeley law-suit revisited, 1417-39', *Southern History* **9**, 1987, 34-50.

SMITH, WILLIAM JAMES. 'The rise of the Berkeleys: an account of the Berkeleys of Berkeley Castle, 1243-1361', *B.G.A.S.Tr.* **70**, 1951, 64-80 and **71**, 1952, 101-21. Includes pedigree, 12-14th c.

Berkeley continued

SMYTH, JOHN. *The Berkeley manuscripts: the lives of the Berkeleys, lords of the Honour, castle and manor of Berkeley, in the County of Gloucester, from 1066 to 1618, with a description of the Hundred of Berkeley and of its inhabitants*, ed., Sir John MacLean. 3 vols. Gloucester: J. Bellows for B.G.A.S., 1883-5. Includes much documentary material.

'The Berkeleys of Uley', *G.N.Q.* **7**, 1900, 127-33, and 153-8. Includes outline pedigree, 11-16th c. See also Barclay.

Berewe
See Paulet.

Bigland
GRAY, IRVINE. 'Ralph Bigland and his family,' *B.G.A.S.Tr.* **75**, 1956, 116-33. Includes pedigree, 17-18th c.

Blagden
See Hale.

Booth
See Annesley.

Boteler
See Sudeley.

Bower
BOWER, HUBERT. *Bower family of Gloucestershire*. [London]: privately published, 1871.

Bradeston
AUSTIN, ROLAND. 'Notes on the family of Bradeston', *B.G.A.S.Tr.* **47**, 1925, 279-86. Medieval.

Bray
BROWNE, A.L. 'The Bray family in Gloucestershire', *B.G.A.S.Tr.* **55**, 1933, 293-315. Includes pedigree, 15-17th c.

BROWNE, A.L. 'The Brays of Great Barrington', *B.G.A.S.Tr.* **57**, 1935, 158-75. 17-18th c.

Britton
STILSBURY, G. BRITTON. *The Brittons of Kingswood Chase and some Gloucestershire connections, 1498-1985*. Bristol: V. Britton, c.1985.

Brooke
BROOKE, GILBERT EDWARD. *Brooke of Horton in the Cotswolds, with notes on some other Brooke families*. Singapore: Methodist Publishing House, 1918. Includes pedigree, 14-19th c.

Family Histories continued

Brown
BELLOWS, JOHN. *Browns of Bartonbury*. Gloucester: John Bellows, 1899. Reprinted from *Friends quarterly examiner*, 7th month, 1899.
HAINES, ROBERT J. 'Has anyone seen Charlie Brown?' *J.G.F.H.S.* **39**, 1988, 15-16. See also **40**, 1989, 12. Brown family, 18-19th c.

Browne
BADDELEY, ST. CLAIR. 'The Brownes of Woodchester and the Roman Pavement', *Notes and queries* **151**, 1926, 94-5. 18th c.
MARSHALL, CHARLES W. *The Browne family of Bristol, London, etc., from the mid-seventeenth century*. Exeter: the author, 1979.

Brydges
BELTZ, GEO. FRED. *Review of the Chandos peerage case, adjudicated 1803, and of the pretensions of Sir Samuel Egerton Brydges, bart., to designate himself per legem terrae Baron Chandos of Sudeley*. R Bentley, 1834. Brydges and Knatchbull families.

Bubb
BUBB, G.W. 'Researching the Bubb family history', *J.G.F.H.S.* **6**, 1980, 10-14. 17-19th c.
PITHER, MAUREEN. 'The Bubb family', *J.G.F.H.S.* **36**, 1988, 13. Births, marriages and deaths, 19th c.

Budgett
LINDEGAARD, PATRICIA. *The Budgetts of Kingswood Hill and their Bristol family*. Brislington: [the author?] 1988. Includes pedigree, 18-19th c.

Busby
STAPLETON, GUY. 'A family in transition: the weaving Busbys of Moreton, Gloucestershire', *Genealogists magazine* **17**, 1972, 67-74. 18-19th c.

Bushell
LANGSTON, J.N. 'Old Catholic families of Gloucestershire: the Bushells of Broad Marston', *B.G.A.S.Tr.* **75**, 1956, 105-15 and 144-1. Includes pedigree, 13-17th c.

Butler
See Little.

Cambray
DUNBAR-DUNBAR, J.A. *Family of Cambray of Great Rissington and Icomb, Gloucestershire, with a note upon the medieval Cambrays*. Phillimore, 1898. Includes pedigrees, 16-20th c., with monumental inscriptions, wills *etc.*

Canning
N. 'The family of Canning', *Herald & Genealogist* **1**, 1863, 273-7. Of Bristol, includes pedigree, 13th c.
WADLEY, T.P. 'The Cannings of Foxcott', *Genealogist* **4**, 1880, 157-65. Of Foxcott, Warwickshire, and Gloucestershire, includes extracts from parish registers.

Canynges
PRYCE, GEORGE. *Memorials of the Canynges family and their times: their claim to be regarded as the founder and restorers of Westbury College and Redcliffe church, critically examined to which is added, inedited memoranda relating to Chatterton*. Bristol: the author, 1854.

Caruthers
See Little.

Cary
HALL, I.V. 'The grant of arms to the Cary family', *B.G.A.S.Tr.* **70**, 1951, 155-6. 1700.
See also Knight.

Cassey
LANGSTON, J.N. 'Old Catholic families of Gloucestershire: the Casseys of Wightfield in Deerhurst.' *B.G.A.S.Tr.* **74**, 1955, 128-52. Includes pedigree, 14-17th c.

Catchmay
ALLEN, WILLIAM TAPNELL. 'The family of Catchmay', *B.G.A.S.Tr.* **24**, 1901, 142-55. 14-18th c., includes extracts from parish registers, monumental inscriptions *etc.*

Challoner
See Knight.

Chandos
See Brydges.

Chatterton
New facts relating to the Chatterton family gathered from manuscript entries in a 'history of the Bible', which once belonged to the parents of Thomas Chatterton the poet, and from parish registers. Bristol: W. George & Son, 1883. 18th c.
See also Canynges.

Family Histories continued

Chester
WATERS, ROBERT EDMOND CHESTER. *Genealogical memoirs of the families of Chester of Bristol, Barton Regis, London and Almondsbury, descended from Henry Chester, sheriff of Bristol 1470, and also of the families of Astry of London, Kent, Beds., Hunts., Oxon. and Gloucestershire descended from Sir Ralph Astry, Kt., Lord Mayor of London, 1493*. Reeves & Turner, 1881.

Clare
ALTSCHUL, MICHAEL. *A baronial family in medieval England: the Clares 1217-1314*. Baltimore: Johns Hopkins Press, 1965.
MACLAGAN, M. 'The heraldry of the house of Clare', *Family history* 2(85/6) N.S., **61/2**, 1981, 2-12. Includes pedigree, 10-14th c.

Cleeveley
PAGET, M. 'A family of craftsmen and husbandmen: the Cleeveleys of Charlton Kings.' *C.K.L.H.S.B.* **11**, 1984, 29-43; **12**, 1984, 36-42; **13**, 1985, 35-47. See also: **15**, 1986, 53-4. Includes pedigree. 16-18th c.

Clifford
CLIFFORD, HUGH. *The house of Clifford from before the conquest*. Phillimore, 1988.
'Pedigree of Clifford of Frampton, Co. Gloucester, of Dublin, and of Castle Annesley, Co. Wexford,' *M.G.H.* series **5**, 5, 1925, 313-25.

Clutterbuck
WITCHELL, MARK EDWIN NORTHAM & HUDLESTON, CHRISTOPHER ROY.ed. *An account of the principal branches of the family of Clutterbuck from the sixteenth century to the present, chiefly based upon the Heralds' visitations*. Gloucester: John Bellows, 1924. Includes pedigrees.
'The Clutterbuck family, of Stanley St Leonards', *G.N.Q.* **3**, 1887, 6-9.
'The family of Clutterbuck', *G.N.Q.* **5**, 1894, 378-93, 426-7, 454-60, 511-13, and 546-60; **6**, 1896, 13-16. Includes pedigrees, 16-19th c.

Coates
See Russell.

Codrington
CODRINGTON, R.H. 'A family connexion of the Codrington family in the XVIIth century', *B.G.A.S.Tr.* **18**, 1893-4, 134-9.
CODRINGTON, R.H. *Memoirs of the family of Codrington of Codrington, Didmarton, Frampton-on-Severn and Dodington*. Letchworth: Arden Press, 1916.

Codrington *continued*
CODRINGTON, R.H. 'Memoirs of the family of Codrington of Codrington, Didmarton, Frampton-on-Severn, and Dodington', *B.G.A.S.Tr.* **21**, 1898, 301-45. Includes pedigrees, 14-19th c.
LOWE, ROBSON. *The Codrington correspondence, 1743-1851*. Robson Lowe, 1951.

Colchester
DIGHTON, CONWAY. 'The Colchester family', *G.N.Q.* **5**, 1894, 251-2. Extracts from Ashleworth parish register.

Collet
CHADD, MARGARET. *The Collet sagas*. Norwich: Elvery Dowers, 1988. Gloucestershire, Suffolk and London.

Cotton
See Annesley.

Cowmeadow
PERRY, DAVID. 'The history and genealogy of the Cowmeadow family', *J.G.F.H.S.* **36**, 1988, 26-8. 16-18th c.

Crossman
HAINES, R.J. 'The Crossmans of Almondsbury', *J.B.A.* **32**, 1983, 11-13. Mainly 17th c.

Crupes
See Scrupes.

Currier
See Batte.

Dadswell
BALCH, BARBARA. *A Dadswell family history and genealogy, c.1560-1980*. London, Ontario: the author, 1980.

Daubeney
GREENFIELD, B.W. 'On the Daubeney family and its connection with Gloucestershire', *B.G.A.S.Tr.* **10**, 1885-6, 175-85. 13-14th c.
HALL, I.V. 'The Daubeney's', *B.G.A.S.Tr.* **84**, 1965, 113-40 and **85**, 1966, 175-201. Includes pedigree, 18-19th c.

Daubrie
BUTTREY, PAM. 'The Daubrie family (four generations) recorded', *J.G.F.H.S.* **36**, 1988, 31-2. 17-18th c.

Daunt
DAUNT, JOHN. 'The Daunt family', *G.N.Q.* **2**, 1884, 286-8. 15-17th c.
DAUNT, JOHN. *Some account of the family of Daunt*. Newcastle-upon-Tyne: J.M. Carr, 1881.

Family Histories continued

Davies
'A Davies bible', *J.G.F.H.S.* **39**, 1988, 19-20. Birth, marriage and death notices in family bible.

Deane
See Dene.

De Chedder
GEORGE, W. 'The De Chedder family of Bristol and Cheddar', *Somerset Archaeological & Natural History Society proceedings*. **34**(2), 1888, 114-6. 13-14th c.

De Havilland
DE HAVILLAND, JOHN VON SONTTAG. *A chronicle of the ancient and noble Norman family of De Havilland, originally of Haverland in the Cotentin, Normandy, now of Guernsey, including the English branches of Havelland of Dorsetshire, also extinct, and Haviland of Somersetshire, with the documentary evidences.* St Louis: Mekeel Press, 1895.

Deighton
DIGHTON, CONWAY. 'The Deightons of Gloucester', *G.N.Q.* **5**, 1894, 135-6. 17th c.
MORIARTY, G. ANDREWS. 'Some notes on Deighton, Gookin, Terrill, and Gifford of Brimpsfield', *B.G.A.S.Tr.* **66**, 1947, 246-54.

De Miners
BADDELEY, ST CLAIR. 'The De Miners family', *Notes & queries,* July 1919, 170-1. 12th c.

Dene
DEANE, MARY. *The book of Dene, Deane, Adeane: a genealogical history.* Elliot Stock, 1899. Includes pedigrees, 16-19th c.

Dimock
FLETCHER, W.G.D. 'Dimock of Randwick and Stonehouse, Co. Gloucester', *Genealogist* **2**, 1878, 181-3. See also **3**, 1879, 326-7. 18-19th c.
FLETCHER, W..G. DIMOCK. 'The Dimocks of Gloucester', *G.N.Q.* **5**, 1894, 269-71. 17-19th c.
FLETCHER, W.G. DIMOCK. 'The family of Dimock, of Randwick and Stonehouse', *G.N.Q.* **5**, 1894, 240-9 and 269-71. Pedigree, 17-19th c.
FLETCHER, W.G. DIMOCK. 'Register extracts relating to the Dimock family', *Genealogist* **2**, 1878, 213-4. 17-18th c.

Dobell
'Detmore and the Dobell family', *C.K.L.H.S.B.* **5**, 1981, 11-29, **6**, 1981, 32-9. Includes pedigree, 18-20th c.

Dorney
'Dorney family: extracts from the Uley registers', *G.N.Q.* **3**, 1887, 440-1.

Dowdeswell
DOWDESWELL, E.R. 'Dowdeswell family', *G.N.Q.* **2**, 1884, 410-12. See also 530-2.

Dudbridge
DUDBRIDGE, BRYAN J. 'The descendants of Joseph Dudbridge the clothier', *J.G.F.H.S.* **39**, 1988, 17-18. 17-20th c.
DUDBRIDGE, B.J. 'The Dudbridge family in Bristol', *J.B.A.* **52**, 1988, 26-31. Mainly 18-19th c., includes pedigree.

Dutton
Historical and genealogical memoirs of the Dutton family of Sherborne, in Gloucestershire, as represented in the peerage of England by the Right Hon. the Baron Sherborne. [ ]: privately printed, 1899. Includes pedigree. 16-18th c.
Memoirs of the Duttons of Dutton in Cheshire, with notes respecting the Sherborne branch of the family. Henry Sotheran & Co., Chester: Marshall & Meeson, 1901. Sherborne, Gloucestershire.

Dymer
See Whitefield.

Eden
BARNARD, E.A.B. *The Edens of Honeybourne, Gloucestershire: an old time correspondence, 1785-1839.* Evesham: W. & H. Smith, 1929.

Edwards
BUTTREY, PAM. 'The Edwards of Hewelsfield and St Briavels', *J.G.F.H.S.* **35**, 1987, 31-2. 18-19th c.

Elton
See Mayo.

Finnimore
PHILLIMORE, W.P.W. 'On the origin of Finnimore and its allied surnames', *G.N.Q.* **2**, 1884, 309-16.

Forster
GOULSTONE, JOHN. 'The Forsters of Bristol and some descendants', *J.B.A.* **58**, 1989, 31-5. Includes pedigree. 12-18th c.

Fortescue
FORTESCUE, THOMAS, LORD CLERMONT. *History of the family of Fortescue in all its branches.* 2nd ed. Ellis & White, 1880.

Family Histories continued

Fowler
FOWLER, W.G., 'The Fowlers of King's Stanley and Stonehouse', *J.B.A.* **10**, 1977, 14-17; **12**, 1978, 23-7; **14**, 1978, 6-10.
'Fowlers of Gloucestershire', *G.N.Q.* **1**, 1881, 223-5, 282-4 and 450-1; **2**, 1884, 55-7, 172-5, 324-6, and 405-9. Includes wills, inquisitions post mortem etc., not completed.

Fox
'Genealogical memoranda relating to the family of Fox, of Brislington, etc.', *M.G.H.*, N.S. **1**, 1894, 114-8 and 283-5. Includes pedigree.

Freeman
DOWDESWELL, E.R. 'Notes on the Freeman family of Bushley, 1620-1700', *G.N.Q.* **3**, 1887, 168-70.
See also Marshall.

Fust
FUST, JENNIFER H. 'Fust family: extracts from Hill registers', *G.N.Q.* **3**, 1887, 587-94.
FUST, JENNIFER H. 'The Fust family portraits', *G.N.Q.* **4**, 1890, 102-27. See also **4**, 201. List of portraits, including much genealogical information, with notes on arms.

Garlick
HALL, I.V. 'The Garlicks, two generations of a Bristol family (1692-1781)', *B.G.A.S.Tr.* **80**, 1961, 132-59. Includes pedigree, 18th c.

Garne
GARNE, RICHARD O. *Cotswold yeomen and sheep: the Garnes of Gloucestershire.* Regency, 1984. Includes pedigrees, 16-20th c.

Gayner
GAYNER, MARGARET. *From Smithy to computer: a history of one Gayner family, 1582-1983.* [ ]: [the author?], 1985. Includes pedigrees.

Gibbes
GIBBS, HENRY HUCKS. 'Pedigree of Gibbes of Bedminster and Bristol, allied to Harington of Kelston, Somerset', *M.G.H.* 2nd series **1**, 1886, 3-6.

Giffard
BAZELEY, WILLIAM. 'Brimpsfield Castle and its owners', *B.G.A.S.Tr.* **20**, 1895-7, 233-40. Giffard family, medieval.
LANGSTON, J.N. 'The Giffards of Brimpsfield', *B.G.A.S.Tr.* **65**, 1944, 105-28. Includes pedigrees, 11-14th c.

Gifford
See Deighton.

Gookin
HUDLESTON, C. ROY. 'Sir Vincent Gookin of Highfield, Gloucestershire', *B.G.A.S.Tr.* **64**, 1943, 113-7. Includes pedigree, 16-17th c., and will, 1638.
See also Deighton.

Gorges
See Knight.

Gostlett
See Hooke.

Gough
MULLIN, DAVID. 'The Gough family of the New Inn, Bream', *New regard* **4**, 1988, 24-34. Includes pedigree. 16-17th c.

Grace
PARKER, GRAHAME. 'The Grace trail', *J.B.A.* **53**, 1988, 26-9. Includes pedigree. 18-20th c.

Graves
MACLEAN, SIR JOHN. 'The family of Graves', *Genealogist* **4**, 1880, 103-6. Grant of arms to Richard Graves of Mickleton, 1728.

Green
BUTTREY, PAM. 'Gloucestershire Greens', *J.G.F.H.S.* **39**, 1988, 13-14. 18-19th c.

Greville
G., I.E. 'The Greville-Tame marriage', *B.G.A.S.Tr.* **76**, 1957, 171-2. c.1501.
PAGET, M. 'The Grevill pedigree', *C.K.L.H.S.B.*, **8**, 1982, 718. 17-18th c.

Guise
DAVIES, G., ed. 'Memoirs of the family of Guise', *Camden third series* **28**, 1917, 83-177. See also index, 178-84. Includes pedigrees, c.15-18th c. of Elmore.
MACLEAN, SIR JOHN. 'Elmore and the Guise family', *B.G.A.S.Tr.* **3**, 1878-9, 49-78. Includes pedigree of Guise, 13-18th c.

Hale
HALE, WILLIAM MATTHEW. *The family of Hale.* [Rake]: privately printed, 1936.
LINDLEY, E.S. 'Hale of Alderley', *B.G.A.S.Tr.* **74**, 1955, 199-202. Includes pedigree of Hale, 16-20th c., and Blagden, 17-19th c.

Hallewell
SANDERS, GEOFFREY. 'The Hallewell family', *B.G.A.S.Tr.* **92**, 1973, 190-97. 19th c.

Family Histories continued

Hamlett
LANE, G.B. 'The Hamlett family', *C.K.L.H.S.B.* **9**, 1989, 38-46. Includes pedigree, 18-20th c.

Harington
'Extracts from the registers of the parishes of Kelston and Corston, Somerset, and from Bitton in Gloucestershire', *M.G.H.*, N.S. **3**, 1880, 194-7. Relating to the Harington family. Many works on this family are listed in the Somerset volume of *British genealogical bibliographies*. See also Gibbes.

Hartland
PAGET, M. 'The Hartland pedigree', *C.K.L.H.S.B.* **7**, 1982, 13-15. 16-19th c.

Haviland
See De Havilland.

Hawthorne
'The Hawthorne family', *C.K.L.H.S.B.* **18**, 1987, 5. Includes pedigree, 16-18th c.

Haynes
POYNTON, F.J. 'The family of Haynes of Westbury-on-Trym, Wick and Abson, and other places in Gloucestershire', *B.G.A.S.Tr.* **9**, 1884-5, 277-97. See also **10**, 1885-6, 226-9. Includes pedigree, 15-18th c., wills, and monumental inscriptions.

Heane
HEANE, WILLIAM C. *Genealogical notes relating to the family of Heane*. Mitchell & Hughes 1887. Originally published *M.G.H.*, 2nd series **2**, 167-8, 180-2, and 209-12. Includes extracts from registers, monumental inscriptions, wills and pedigree, 17-19th c.
HEANE, WILLIAM C. 'The Heane family', *G.N.Q.* **3**, 1887, 232-3. Parish register extracts.

Hearne
See Martyn.

Hicks
HICKS BEACH, MRS WILLIAM. *A Cotswold family: Hicks and Hicks Beach*. William Heinemann, 1909. 16-19th c.
POYNTON, FRANCIS J. 'A doubtful point in the genealogy of Hicks of Beverston as it appears in Burke's peerage and baronage', *B.G.A.S.Tr.* **11**, 1886-7, 260-5. Includes pedigree, 17-19th c.
'Some account of the later Hicks's of Stinchcombe', *G.N.Q.* **10**(87), 1913, 1-9.

Hillier
HORTON-SMITH, L.G.H. 'The Hillier family of Cirencester from 1635 together with the family of Parry, and supplement', *B.G.A.S.Tr.* **64**, 1943, 211-39. 17-20th c.

Hine
See Lane.

Hodges
'The Hodges family of Shipton Moyne', *G.N.Q.* **1**, 1881, 360-3. See also **1**, 455-7, for wills, monumental inscriptions *etc.*, and **2**, 1884, 27. 17th c.

Holbrow
PHILLIMORE, W.P.W. *Some account of the family of Holbrow, of Kingscote, Uley and Leonard Stanley in Gloucestershire*. Phillimore & Co., 1901.

Holder
See Berkeley.

Hooke
TODD, FREDERICK W. *Humphrey Hooke of Bristol and his family and descendants in England and America during the seventeenth century*. New Haven: Tuttle, Morehouse & Taylor, 1938. Includes pedigree of Hooke, 15-17th c., also of Young 15-17th c., Gostlett, 16-17th c., and Scrope of Oxfordshire, 16-17th c., with Hooke wills, *etc.*

Hopkins
BRADENEY, JOSEPH ALFRED. *Genealogical memoranda relating to the families of Hopkins of Llanfihangel Ystern Llewern, Co. Monmouth, and Probyn of Newland, Co. Gloucester*. Mitchell & Hughes, 1889. Includes pedigree, 17-18th c., parish register extracts *etc.*

Howard
See Stafford.

Hungerford
WILMOT, E.A. EARDLEY. 'The Hungerford family of Windrush', *G.N.Q.*, **1**, 1881, 272-3. 16-18th c.

Hutchyns
See Tyndale.

Jacobs
JOSEPH, Z. 'The Jacobs of Bristol, glassmakers to King George III', *B.G.A.S.Tr.* **95**, 1977, 98-101. 18-19th c.

Jenkinson
DENNY, HENRY LYTTLETON LYSTER. *The manor of Hawkesbury and its owners*. Gloucester: J. Bellows, 1920. Jenkinson family, 16-20th c., includes pedigree.

Family Histories continued

Jenner
FYNMORE, R.J. 'Jenner, of Gloucestershire and Wiltshire', *G.N.Q.* **10**, 1914, 49-59. Includes pedigree, 18-19th c.

Jennings
See Knight.

Jerningham
BERGIN, MICHAEL. 'The Jerninghams and Painswick,' *Gloucestershire & North Avon Catholic History Society Journal* **15**, 1990, 2-7. 16-19th c.
LANGSTON, J.N. 'The Jerninghams of Painswick,' *B.G.A.S.Tr.* **83**, 1964, 99-118. 16-18th c.

Johnson
MONEY, WALTER. 'The family of James Johnson, successively Bishop of Gloucester and Worcester,' *B.G.A.S.Tr.* **8**, 1883-4, 324-41. Includes pedigree, 17-19th c., with monumental inscriptions.
MONEY, WALTER. 'The family of James Johnson, successively Bishop of Gloucester and Worcester', *B.G.A.S.Tr.* **9**, 1884-5, 356-7. Pedigrees of American branch of the family, 18th c.

Jones
See Matthews.

Jordan
SALE, J. 'The Jordan family of Withy Holt', *C.K.L.H.S.B.* **20**, 1988, 37-9. 19-20th c.

Kent
KENT, GEORGE. *The Kents on the hop, 1381-1989: a family story.* Cambridge: the author, 1989. Gloucestershire family.

Kerr
KERR, RUSSELL J. *A history of the family of Kerr, of the House, Newnham, Gloucestershire, which is descended from the houses of Ferniehurst and of Ancrum.* Gloucester: John Bellows, 1923.

Kingscote
POTTER, ARTHUR KINGSCOTE. 'The Kingscote of Kingscote', *Local history bulletin* **49**, 1984, 3-6. Brief note, 12-19th c.
See also Berkeley.

Knatchbull
See Brydges.

Knight
HALL, I.V. 'The connexions between John Knight, Junior, and the Jennings, Latch and Gorges families, 1641-1653', *B.G.A.S.Tr.* **74**, 1955, 188-99.
HALL, I.V. 'The connexions between John Knight, Jnr., and the Parsons and Jennings families, 1641-79', *B.G.A.S.Tr.* **70**, 1951, 119-25.
HALL, I.V. 'John Knight Junior, sugar refiner at the Great House on St. Augustine's Back (1654-1679): Bristol's second sugar house', *B.G.A.S.Tr.* **68**, 1949, 110-64. Includes pedigrees of Challoner, Knight and Cary, 16-17th c.

Lane
HALL, I.V. 'Temple St. Sugar House under the first partnership of Richard Lane and John Hine (1662-78)', *B.G.A.S.Tr.* **76**, 1957, 118-40. Includes pedigrees of Lane, 16-18th c., and Hine, 17-18th c.

Langley
COSS, PETER R. *The Langley family and its cartulary: a study in late medieval 'gentry'.* Dugdale Society occasional papers **22**. Stratford upon Avon: the Society, 1974. Includes pedigree, 13-15th c., of Warwickshire and Gloucestershire.

Latch
See Knight.

Lawrence
LAWRENCE, RICHARD GWYNNE. 'The Lawrence family, of Bourton on the Water', *G.N.Q.* **2**, 1884, 15-17. 17-18th c.
See also Paulet.

Leigh
DENNISON, SHEILA. 'Nympsfield and the Leigh family', *Gloucestershire & North Avon Catholic History Society Journal* **13**, 1990, 4-13. 19-20th c.

Little
LITTLE, E. CARUTHERS. *Our family history.* Gloucester: John Bellows, 1892. Little family: includes notes on Palling, Carruthers, Butler and White families.

Longden
LONGDEN, H. ISHAM. 'Longden family of Gloucester', *G.N.Q.* **3**, 1887, 36-7, 214-6, and 244-6.
LONGDEN, H. ISHAM. 'The family of Longden', *G.N.Q.* **5**, 1894, 230-33. 17-18th c.

Family Histories continued

Longe
DIGHTON, CONWAY. 'Longe of Ashelworth', *G.N.Q.* **10**, 1904, 22-6. Extracts from the parish register, 1566-1674.

Ludlow
MAYO, C.H. 'Ludlow of Chipping Sodbury', *G.N.Q.* **5**, 1894, 443-5. Includes extracts from parish registers *etc.*

Lyne
LYNE, ROBT. EDWIN. 'The Lyne family, of Little Compton', *G.N.Q.* **2**, 1884, 34-7.

Lysons
GLOCESTRIENSIS. 'The Lysons family', *G.N.Q.* **2**, 1884, 533-5.
GRAY, IRVINE. 'The Lysons family', *B.G.A.S.Tr.* **81**, 1962, 212-3. Includes pedigrees, 16-20th c.
MESSAM, W. 'The Lysons family connection with Rodmarton', *Local History bulletin* **39** (actually **41**), 1980, 5-8. 18-19th c.

Mace
MACE, CHARLES A. 'Mace family', *Notes & queries*, 12th series **11**, 1922, 156-7. See also **150**, 1926, 410. Parish register extracts.

Machen
MACHEN, H.A. 'The Machen family, Gloucestershire', *B.G.A.S.Tr.* **64**, 1943, 96-112. Includes pedigree, 16-20th c.

Makeig
BAYLISS, W.J. 'The Makeigs of Cardigan: Bristol fashion', *J.B.A.* **5**, 1976, 23-6; **6**, 1977, 22-4; **7**, 1977, 12-14. Of Cardigan and Bristol; 18-19th c.

Marisall
MARSHALL, GEORGE W. 'The Marisall family', *G.N.Q.* **1**, 1881, 74-80.

Marshall
MARSHALL, GEORGE W. 'Marshall of Selaby, Co. Durham and Freeman of Batsford, Co. Gloucester', *G.N.Q.* **1**, 1881, 131-5. 17-18th c.

Martin
HUDLESTON, C. ROY. 'The Martins of Redland Court, Bristol', *B.G.A.S.Tr.* **56**, 1934, 83-93. Includes pedigree. 17-18th c.

Martyn
WHITAKER, J. 'The Martyns and the Hearnes: recollections of a grandson', *C.K.L.H.S.B.* **22**, 1989, 16-26.

Matthews
GRAY, IRVINE. 'Records of four Tewkesbury vicars, *c*.1685-1769', *B.G.A.S.Tr.* **102**, 1984, 155-72. Matthews and Jones families, 18th c.

Mayo
MAYO, C.H. *A genealogical account of the Mayo and Elton families of Wilts. and Hereford and some other adjoining counties, to which are added many genealogies ... of families allied by marriage to the family of Mayo, and a history of the manors of Andrewes and Le Mote, in Cheshunt, Hertfordshire.* 2nd ed. 1908. Mayo of Wiltshire, Dorset, Gloucestershire and Herefordshire, Elton of Herefordshire.

Monoux
BOSWORTH, GEORGE F., & SAUNDERS, CONSTANCE DERRAIN., ed. *Original documents relating to the Monoux family.* Walthamstow Antiquarian Society official publications **19**. Walthamstow: the Society, 1928. Of Walthamstow, Essex, London, Gloucestershire and Worcestershire. Includes deeds, inquisitions post mortem, wills *etc.*

Moore
MOORE, D.T. 'The descendants of John Lawrence Moore (1779-1854) of Bristol: carver, gilder and picture frame maker', *J.B.A.* **17**, 1979, 5-9.

Muchgros
MOUGHTON, F.T.S. 'Family of Muchgros', *Birmingham Archaeological Society transactions* **47**, 1921, 8-34. Of Gloucestershire, Somerset and various other counties, 11-13th c.

Oldisworth
WADLEY, THOMAS 'Oldisworth family', *G.N.Q.* **4**, 1890, 556-7. Extracts from Bourton on the Hill parish register, 1606-78.

Oliver
OLIVER, V.L. 'The Oliver family', *G.N.Q.* **5**, 1894, 155-60. See also 322-5. 18th c. pedigree.

Osborne
LINGEN-WATSON, A. 'Fathers-in-law: the Osbornes and Seagers, Bristol solicitors', *J.B.A.* **15**, 1979, 9-10. 18th c.

Overbury
MARSHALL, G.W. 'The Overbury family', *Genealogist* **1**, 1877, 267-70. See also **2**, 1878, 364-5. Continuation of notes previously published in the *Herald & genealogist.* Includes will of Sir Nicholas Overbury of Bourton on the Hill, 1640, with extracts from London parish registers, 16-17th c.

Family Histories continued

Overbury *continued*
'Pedigree of Overbury', *Genealogist* **1**, 1877, 271-6. Of Gloucestershire and Warwickshire, 16-17th c.

Palling
See Little.

Parker
PARKER, EDWARD MILWARD SEEDE. *Genealogical memoranda relating to the family of Parker, of Upton House, Upton Cheyney Manor, Bitton, Gloucestershire, and Welford House, Keynsham, Somerset, of Henbury, Clifton, Bristol, London and elsewhere, from 1543 to 1898.* Bristol: Lavars & Co., 1899. See also Paulet.

Parry
See Hillier and Knight.

Parsons
See Knight.

Paston
LANGSTON, J.N. 'The Pastons of Horton', *B.G.A.S.Tr.* **77**, 1958, 97-126. Includes pedigree, 15-19th c.

Paul
HYETT, SIR FRANCIS. 'Sir George Onesiphorus Paul', *B.G.A.S.Tr.* **51**, 1929, 143-68. Includes pedigree, 17-19th c.

Paulet
FRANKLYN, CHARLES A.H. *A genealogical history of the families of Paulet (or Pawlett), Berewe (or Barrow) Lawrence and Parker ...* Bedford: Foundry Press, 1963. Paulet of Gloucestershire, Barrow of Gloucestershire, Lawrence of Lancashire and Gloucestershire, Parker of Glamorganshire and Monmouthshire.

Pauncefote
DIGHTON, CONWAY. 'The Pauncefote family', *G.N.Q.* **5**, 1894, 268-9. Extracts from Ashleworth parish register.
LANGSTON, J.N. 'Old Catholic families of Gloucestershire I: The Pauncefotes of Hasfield', *B.G.A.S.Tr.* **71**, 1952, 122-44. See also **73**, 1954, 235-6.

Phelps
TANN, JENNIFER. 'Some account books of the Phelps family of Dursley', *B.G.A.S.Tr.* **86**, 1967, 107-17. General discussion with list of 18th c. clothiers.

Phillipps
MUNBY, A.N.L. *The family affairs of Sir Thomas Phillipps.* Phillipps studies **2**. Cambridge: C.U.P., 1952.

Pillinger
LINDEGAARD, PATRICIA. 'Extracts from the visiting book of the Rev Charles Parkin, curate of Brislington, 1827', *J.B.A.* **8**, 1977, 5-6. Notes on various Pillinger families.

Pope
HALL, IVY. 'Whitson Court Sugar House, Bristol', *B.G.A.S.Tr.* **65**, 1944, 1-97. Pope family, includes pedigree, 17-19th c.

Poyntz
MACLEAN, SIR JOHN. *Historical and genealogical memoirs of the family of Poyntz, or, eight centuries of an English house.* Exeter: William Pollard, 1886. Includes pedigrees.
THOMPSON, H.L. 'The Poyntz family', *B.G.A.S.Tr.* **4**, 1879-80, 73-85.

Probyn
See Hopkins.

Robin
G., J. 'The Robin family: Gloucestershire', *G.N.Q.* **4**, 1890, 159-62. 16-18th c.

Robinson
DARWIN, BERNARD. *Robinsons of Bristol, 1844-1944.* Bristol: E.S. & A. Robinson, 1945.

Rooke
WAGNER, HENRY. 'Pedigree of Rooke, of Co's Kent and Gloucestershire', *Genealogist* **4**, 1880, 195-208. 16-19th c., includes wills, extracts from parish registers, and monumental inscriptions.

Rowlands
ROWLANDS, ELISABETH. *John and Annie Rowlands and their family.* Cheltenham: the author, 1985.

Rudder
PHILLIMORE, W.P.W. 'The Rudder family', *G.N.Q.* **2**, 1884, 80-82. 17-18th c.

Russell
TRATEBAS, GLADYS N. 'Russell and Coates family of Cheltenham and London', *J.G.F.H.S.* **38**, 1988, 22-3. Includes pedigree, 19th c.

Sargent
SARGEAUNT, W.T. 'Sargent of Gloucester, U.S.A.', *B.G.A.S.Tr.* **85**, 1966, 224-6. 17th c.
SARGEAUNT, W.T. 'The family of Sargeaunt of Hart Barn, Longhope', *B.G.A.S.Tr.* **78**, 1959, 110-17. Includes pedigree, 16-20th c., with will of William Sargent, 1568/9.

Family Histories continued

Scrope
See Hooke.

Scrupes
CLAY, C.T. 'The family of Scrupes or Crupes of Whittington, Gloucestershire', *B.G.A.S.Tr.* **65**, 1944, 129-40.

Seager
See Osborne.

Selwyn
BAZELEY, WILLIAM. 'Some records of Motson in the County of Gloucester, and of the Selwyns', *B.G.A.S.Tr.* **2**, 1877/8, 241-84. Includes pedigrees of Selwyn of Sussex and Gloucestershire, 15-19th c.
SWYNNERTON, CHARLES. 'Some early Selwyns', *B.G.A.S.Tr.* **47**, 1925, 205-9. Medieval.

Sheppard
BODDINGTON, R.S. *Pedigree of the family of Sheppard*, privately published, 1883.
SHEPPARD, WILLIAM ALBERT. *A brief history of the Sheppard family, formerly seated at the manors of Avening, Minchinhampton, and Colesbourne ... with pedigrees of the elder and junior branches of these ancient families ...* Calcutta: privately printed, 1891.

Sherborne
See Dutton.

Shipway
HAINES, ROBERT J. 'The Shipway pedigree fraud, or, Regina v. Davies, 1897', *Gloucestershire History* **4**, 1990, 5-6.
PHILLIMORE, W.P.W. *The 'principal genealogical specialist', or, Regina v. Davies and the Shipway genealogy, being the story of a remarkable pedigree fraud.* Phillimore & Co., 1899.

Slaughter
'The Slaughter family', *G.N.Q.* **2**, 1884, 64-8. See also **17**.

Smyth
The Smyths of Ashton Court were originally a Gloucestershire family, and retained their Bristol connections even though their residence, Ashton Court, was actually in Somerset. Hence works on them are listed here.
BANTOCK, ANTON. *The earlier Smyths of Ashton Court from their letters 1545-1741.* Bristol: Malago Society, 1982. Includes pedigree.

Smyth continued

BANTOCK, ANTON. *The inside story of the Smyths of Ashton Court.* Bristol: Malago Archives Committee, 1977.
BANTOCK, ANTON. *The later Smyths of Ashton Court from their letters, 1741-1802.* Bristol: Malago Society, 1984.
BANTOCK, ANTON. *The last Smyths of Ashton Court, Pt.1. 1802-1860.* Bristol: Malago Society, 1980.
BETTEY, J.H. *The rise of a gentry family: the Smyths of Ashton Court, c.1500-1642.* Bristol: Historical Association, 1978.
PINK, W.D. 'The Smyths of Nibley', *G.N.Q.* **5**, 1894, 420-22. American branch of the family.
WAY, LEWIS UPTON. 'The Smyths of Ashton Court', *B.G.A.S.Tr.*, **31**, 1908, 244-60. Includes list of Bristol merchants, 16th c.

Stafford
JEFFCOAT, R. 'Arms and badges of Edward Stafford, third Duke of Buckingham', *B.G.A.S.Tr.* **54**, 1932, 133-6.
LANGSTON, J.N. 'Old Catholic families of Gloucestershire, II: the Staffords and Howards of Thornbury', *B.G.A.S.Tr.* **72**, 1953, 79-104. Includes pedigree. 14-18th c.

Stephens
DAVIES, W.H. SILVESTER. 'Notes on Chavenage and the Stephens family', *B.G.A.S.Tr.* **22**, 1899, 128-37. Includes pedigree. 16-19th c.

Stiff
PHILLIMORE, W.P.W. 'The Stiff family', *G.N.Q.* **2**, 1884, 614-22. 16-19th c.
'Medieval Stiffs of Hawkesbury', *G.N.Q.* **5**, 1894, 273-83, and 463-76. Includes pedigree.
'On the origin of the surname of Stiff', *G.N.Q.*, **5**, 1894, 113-22, 178-85, and 249-51.

Stokes
SCHOMBERG, ARTHUR. *Some notes of the Stokes family (Cos. Wilts. and Glos.).* Devizes: Gazette Printing Works, 1909. Reprinted from *Wiltshire notes & queries.*

Sturge
GOODBODY, MARGARET. *Five daughters in search of learning: the Sturge family, 1820-1944.* Bristol: M. Goodbody, 1986.

Sudeley
SUDELEY, LORD, & WINKLESS, D. 'Medieval Sudeley', *Family history* **10**(61/2), N.S. **37/8**, 1977, 9-39. Sudeley and Boteler families.

Family Histories continued

Tame
HOLT, HENRY F. 'The Tames of Fairford', *Journal of the British Archaeological Association* **27**, 1871, 110-48. Includes pedigree, 15-16th c. See also Greville.

Teague
ANSTIS, RALPH. *The industrial Teagues and the Forest of Dean*. Gloucester: Alan Sutton, 1990. 18-19th c.

Terrill
See Deighton.

Throckmorton
BIDDLE, DANIEL. 'Some account of the Throckmortons of Tortworth, and a few of their ancestors in other lives', *G.N.Q.* **10**, 1914, 65-72.
MACLEAN, SIR JOHN. 'Pedigree of Throckmorton of Tortworth and Clowerwall', *B.G.A.S.Tr.* **7**, 1882-3, 194. 17th c.

Tippett
'Julia Tippett's family', *J.G.F.H.S.* **7**, 1980, 10. Pedigree, 17-19th c.

Todeni
BROWNE, A.L. 'Robert de Todeni and his heirs', *B.G.A.S.Tr.* **52**, 1920, 103-11. Medieval.

Tombs
'The Tombs of the Cotswolds', *J.G.F.H.S.* **38**, 1988, 15. Tombs family, 18-19th c.

Tomes
'The Tomes family of Marston Sicca', *G.N.Q.* **1**, 1881, 194-5. 14-15th c.

Tracy
SUDELEY, LORD. 'Becket's murderer: William de Tracy', *Family history* **13**(97), 1983, 3-36. Includes notes on the Tracy family of Toddington.
SUDELEY, LORD. 'Toddington and the Tracys', *B.G.A.S.Tr.* **88**, 1969, 127-72. See also **90**, 1971, 216-9. 12-19th c., includes medieval pedigree.
SUDELEY, LORD. 'Toddington and the Tracys', *Local history bulletin* **32**, 1975, 3-5, and **33**, 1976, 4-5. Brief notes. 11-20th c.

Trotman
TROTMAN, F.H. *The Trotman family, 1086 to 1963*. Nottingham: the author, 1965. Includes pedigrees.

Trotman *continued*
PHILLIMORE, W.P.W. 'The Trotman family', *G.N.Q.* **2**, 1884, 201-12. See also 341-6 and 429. 16-19th c.
'Notes on the Trotman family', *G.N.Q.* **5**, 1894, 14-28, 76-84, 122-5, 195-209, 234-40, 283-300 and 334-44. See also 493. Includes many extracts from Cam, Dursley, Syston, and other parish registers, and from wills, monumental inscriptions *etc*.

Twining
TWINING, STEPHEN H. *Some account of an early Twining pedigree and of other references to the name in the fourteenth and fifteenth centuries*. McCorquodale & Co., 1927.

Tyler
The family history of Tyler of Gloucestershire and Bristol. Colchester: E.W. Cullingford & Co., 1913.

Tyndale
COOKE, JAMES HERBERT. 'The Tyndales in Gloucestershire', *B.G.A.S.Tr.* **2**, 1877-8, 29-46. 15-18th c.
GREENFIELD, B.W. 'Notes relating to the family of Tyndale, of Stinchcombe and Nibley in Gloucestershire, the result of an attempt to discover the parentage of William Tyndale alias Hutchyns the martyr', *Genealogist* **2**, 1878, 1-7, 38-43, 123-8, 159-62, 227-30, 319-26, 356-63 and 369-71. See also 68. 15-16th c.
GREENFIELD, B.W. 'Pedigree of the family of Tyndale of Stinchcombe and Nibley, Co. Gloucester', *Genealogist* **2**, 1878, 373-8. 16-19th c.
OVERY, CHARLES & TYNDALE, ARTHUR C. 'The parentage of William Tyndale, alias Hutchyns, Translator and Martyr', *B.G.A.S.Tr.* **73**, 1954, 208-15. 14-16th c.
See also Annesley.

Walcot
WALCOT, M.G. & J. *The Walcots of Birmingham and Bristol: an account of a cadet branch of the ancient family of Walcot of Walcot and Bitterley Court, Shropshire*. Sutton Coldfield: the authors, 1975.

Washbourne
DAVENPORT, JAMES. *The Washbourne family of Little Washbourne and Wichenford in the county of Worcester*. Methuen & Co., 1907.

Weight
H., A.W.C. 'The Weights of Clingre', *G.N.Q.* **6**, 1896, 63-5. 17-19th c.

Family Histories continued

White
See Little.

Whitefield
HUDLESTON, C. ROY. 'George Whitefield's ancestry', *B.G.A.S.Tr.* **59**, 1937, 221-42. Includes pedigrees of Whitefield and Dymer, 17-18th c., with will abstracts.

Whitson
LATIMER, JOHN. 'The alleged arms of John Whitson', *Proceedings of the Clifton Antiquarian Club* **5**, 1900-3, 268-76.

Whittington
BUSH, THOS. S. 'Whittington of Cold Ashton', *G.N.Q.* **6**, 1896, 121-5. Parish register extracts.

WHITTINGTON, MICHAEL. *The Whittington story: from the three counties to the City*. Cirencester: the author, c.1988. Of Herefordshire, Gloucestershire, Worcestershire and London. Includes pedigree.

Willets
'The Willets, or Willett, family', *G.N.Q.* **2**, 1884, 558-61. 16-18th c.

Williams
'The family of Williams of Wotton under Edge', *G.N.Q.* **5**, 1884, 92-6.

Wills
TILL, ROGER. *Wills of Bristol*. [ ]: [Imperial Tobacco Co.], [19..]. W.D. & H.O. Wills Co. Ltd., includes pedigree of family, 18-20th c.

Wood
WOOD, J.C. NEVILLE. 'Proving paternity without an entry of baptism', *Oxfordshire Family Historian*, 1982, **2**(7), 221-23. Wood of Painswick, 18th c.

Woodroffe
Pedigree of Woodroffe of Plusterwine, Co. Gloucester. Mitchell & Hughes, 1876. 15-19th c.

Wynter
RENDELL, BRYAN, [ed.] *The Wynter family: (a collective research)*. Lydney: Whitecross School, 1988. 16-19th c.

RENDELL, B. *Wyntours of the White Cross: an extended family history*. White Cross: White Cross School, 1987.

Wyrall
HILL, MAY C. 'Wyrall lands and deeds', *B.G.A.S.Tr.* **63**, 1942, 190-206. Wyrall family, 17-19th c.

Yeend
W., H. 'Yeend family', *G.N.Q.* **8**, 1900, 15-17. See also 33. Pedigree, 18th c.

Yescombe
YESCOMBE, E.R. 'The Yescombe family', *J.B.A.* **37**, 1984, 15-19. 18th c.

Young
MACLEAN, SIR JOHN. 'Notes on the family of Yonge, or Young, of Bristol, and on the Red Lodge', *B.G.A.S.Tr.* **15**, 1890-1, 227-45. Includes pedigree, 14-17th c.

See also Hooke.

8. PARISH REGISTERS AND OTHER RECORDS OF BIRTHS, MARRIAGES AND DEATHS

The importance of parish registers and other sources of information on births, marriages and deaths cannot be overstated. Genealogists in Gloucestershire and Bristol are fortunate that many registers have been published, in whole or in part. They are less fortunate in that there are no up to date lists of manuscript parish registers. The most recent lists are:

STEEL, D.J. *National index of parish registers: a guide to Anglican, Roman Catholic and Nonconformist registers before 1837, together with information on marriage licences, bishop's transcripts and modern copies*, **5**, South Midlands and Welsh Border, comprising the counties of Gloucestershire, Herefordshire, Oxfordshire, Shropshire, Warwickshire and Worcestershire. Society of Genealogists, 1966 (reprinted Phillimore, 1971).

Diocese of Gloucester: list of bishop's transcripts 1569-1812. Local history pamphlet **5**. Gloucester: Gloucester City Libraries, c.1968. Reprinted from *Catalogue of the Gloucester Diocesan records*.

See also:
RICHARDS' *Handlist*, page 9, above, and
ANTIQUARIUS 'Burn's references to Gloucestershire parish registers', *G.N.Q.* **2**, 1884, 159-62.
CHAPMAN, M.C. 'Parish records transcribed by Roe (marriages)', *J.G.F.H.S.* **6**, 1980, 28-9. List of ms. transcripts at Gloucestershire Record Office.
STONE, B.G. 'Missing registers at Bristol Register Office', *J.B.A.* **49**, 1987, 36-8. List.
'Bristol and Avon marriage indexes', *J.B.A.* **44**, 1986, 13-17. List of registers for which the Bristol & Avon F.H.S. hold indexes, including parishes in South Gloucestershire, Bristol and North Somerset.
'Gloucestershire parish registers', G.N.Q. **1**, 1881, 185-7, **3**, 1887, 97-116; **6**, 1896, 56-61; **9**, 1902, 105-6 and 164-75. Includes list of registers, showing dates of commencement, with some extracts from Quedgeley.
'Parish registers in Bristol Record Office', *J.B.A.* **8**, 1977, 4.

Some 17th c. marriage bonds and allegations have been published, and should be consulted:
FRITH, BRIAN, ed. *Gloucestershire marriage allegations, 1637-1680, with surrogate allegations to 1694*. B.G.A.S. Records branch **2**. Bristol: the Society, 1954.

Continued by:
FRITH, BRIAN, ed. *Marriage allegations in the Diocese of Gloucester*, **2**: 1681-1700. B.G.A.S. Records branch **9**. Bristol: the Society, 1970.
See also:
RALPH, ELIZABETH, ed. *Marriage bonds for the diocese of Bristol excluding the archdeaconry of Dorset*. B.G.A.S. Records branch **1**. Bristol: the Society, 1952. **1**: 1637-1700.
FRY, E.A. ed. *Bristol marriage bonds and allegations, 1660-1684*. Supplement to *G.N.Q.* **85-90**, 1904-14. Originally intended to cover 1637-1799, but *G.N.Q.* ceased publication.

Births, marriages and deaths are frequently recorded in places such as family bibles, newspapers *etc*. See:
HIPWELL, DANIEL. 'Memoranda from an old prayer book', *G.N.Q.* **5**, 1894, 192-4. Births, marriages and deaths, mainly Gloucestershire.
KILLON, M.R. '[List of Gloucestershire parents in nonconformist registers of Dr. Williams' Library at the Public Record Office, 1820-37]', *J.G.F.H.S.* **28**, 1986, 21-22. Letter to the editor; continued in: KILLON, M.R. 'More from Dr. Williams' Library', *J.G.F.H.S.* **29**, 1986, 9-11.
See also:
'It's surprising what you find if you look!', *J.G.F.H.S.* **32**, 1987, 16-18. 18-19th c.
LINDEGAARD, PATRICIA. 'Deaths at sea from Bristol newspapers', *J.B.A.* **47**, 1987, 38. In 1844-5 and 1855.
MOORE, JOHN. 'Extracts from the *Monthly miscellany* for the year 1774', *G.N.Q.* **4**, 1890, 275-9. Gloucestershire marriages, deaths, and ecclesiastical preferments.
P., F. 'Gloucestershire marriages 1774-1776', *G.N.Q.* **5**, 1894, 429-30. From the *Universal magazine*.
SAUL, NIGEL. 'The religious sympathies of the gentry in Gloucestershire', *B.G.A.S.Tr.* **98**, 1980, 99-112. Includes list of burial places of Gloucestershire knights and esquires, 1200-1500.
'Some Gloucestershire marriages, 1733-1736', *G.N.Q.* **1**, 1881, 216-7 and 285-6. Lists marriages, with dowries.

Parish Registers etc. continued

Many Gloucestershire individuals were baptised, married, or buried beyond the county boundary. Numerous lists of 'strays' have been published, especially in *J.B.A.* and *J.G.F.H.S.* The following list is representative rather than comprehensive, and a search through the two journals just mentioned is recommended.

Derbyshire
'Gloucestershire strays in the Derbyshire marriage index', *J.G.F.H.S.* **16**, 1983, 15-16.

Dorset: *Wyke Regis*
'Gloucestershire strays', *J.G.F.H.S.* **6**, 1980, 31. Marriages from Wyke Regis, Dorset, 1795-8.

London and Middlesex: *Westminster*
D., B.C. 'Gloucestershire baptisms at Westminster, 1626-1845', *G.N.Q.* **8**, 1901, 41-4.
D., B.C. 'Gloucestershire burials in Westminster Abbey, 1606-1846', *G.N.Q.* **8**, 1901, 71-88. Includes genealogical notes.
D., B.C. 'Westminster Abbey registers and Gloucestershire', *G.N.Q.* **6**, 1896, 82-4; **8**, 1901, 22-5, 41-4 and 71-88. Extracts, 1655-1746, including much genealogical information.

Oxfordshire
'Gloucestershire marriages in Oxfordshire', *J.G.F.H.S.* **11**, 1981, 26-7. Mainly at Banbury.
'Gloucestershire strays in Oxfordshire', *J.G.F.H.S.* **10**, 1981, 26-8. At Swinbrook, Eynsham, Oxford *etc.*
'Strays', *J.G.F.H.S.* **23**, 1984, 22-5, and **24**, 1985, 17-20. From Oxfordshire.

Sussex: *Brighton*
'East Sussex C.R.O., Lewes: parish register of St. Nicholas, Brighthelmstone [Brighton],: marriages of South Glos. militiamen', *J.G.F.H.S.* **40**, 1989, 26; **41**, 1989, 28. See also **42**, 1989, 11. 1800-1809.

Wiltshire: *Tytherton*
'Strays: registers of Tytherton Moravian Church, Wiltshire', *J.B.A.* **49**, 1987, 21-4. Bristol and Gloucestershire strays.

Worcestershire: *Worcester, Bedwardine*
'Gloucestershire strays from Worcestershire: marriages', *J.G.F.H.S.* **12**, 1982, 26-7. From registers of Worcester and Bedwardine.
'Worcester Cathedral registers (1693-1811): Gloucestershire marriages', *J.G.F.H.S.* **7**, 1980, 26-7.

Numerous Gloucestershire parish registers have been published, especially in *G.P.R.M.* and *G.N.Q.*, although unfortunately the latter often published only extracts rather than full transcripts. Also noted here are notes and general discussions relating to particular registers. The Gloucestershire Family History Society is responsible for:

GLOUCESTERSHIRE FAMILY HISTORY SOCIETY. *Diocese of Gloucester: marriages 1800-1837.* 14 vols. [ ]: G.F.H.S., 1981-6.
1. Abenhall, Blaisdon, Flaxley, Longhope.
2. Lassington, Oxenhall, Pauntley, Rudford, Taynton, Tibberton, Upleadon, Staunton.
3. Upton St. Leonards, Walton Cardiffe, Great Washbourne, Welford, Westcote, Weston Subedge, Weston upon Avon, Whittington, Widford (now Oxon.), Willersey, Winchcombe, Windrush, Winson, Great Witcombe, Withington, Woolstone, Wormington, Yarworth.
4. Adlestrop, Alderton, Aldsworth, Ampney, Ashleworth, Ashton under Hill, Aston Somerville, Aston Subedge, Radgeworth, Bagendon, Barnsley.
5. Barnwood, Great Barrington, Little Barrington, Batsford, Baunton, Beckford, Bibury, Bishops Cleeve, Bisley.
6. Bledington, Boddington, Bourton on the Hill, Brimpsfield, Broadwell, Brockworth, Bromsberrow, Buckland, North Cerney, South Cerney, Charlton Abbotts, Charlton Kings, Chedworth.
7. Cheltenham.
8. Cherington, Childswickham, Churchdown, Clifford Chambers, Coates, Coberley, Cold Aston, Colesbourne, Coln Rogers, Coln St. Aldwyn, Coln St. Dennis, Compton Abdale, Little Compton, Condicote, Corse, Cowley, Cranham, Cutsdean.
9. Daglingworth, Deerhurst, Didbrook, Dorrington, Dowdeswell, Down Hatherley, Driffield, Dumbleton, Dymock, Eastleach Martin, Eastleach Turville, Ebrington, Edgeworth, Elkstone, Elmstone Hardwicke, English Bicknor, Evenlode.
10. Farmington, Flaxley, Forthampton, Guiting Power, Guiting Temple, Hailes, Hampnett, Haresfield, Harnhill, Hartpury, Hasfield, Hawling, Hazelton, Hempstead, Hewelsfield, Hinton on the Green.
11. Gloucester: Christ Church, St. Aldate, St. John the Baptist, St. Mary de Crypt, St. Michaels.
12. Quenington, Quinton, Randwick, Redmarley, Rendcombe, Rodmarton, Ruardean, St. Briavels, Saintbury, Salperton, Sandhurst, Sapperton.

Parish Registers etc. continued

13. Long Marston, Matson, Mickleton, Miserden, Mitcheldean, Moreton in Marsh, Naunton, Newent, Newland.
14. Northleach, Norton, Notgrove, Oddington, Oxenton, Painswick, Pebworth, Pitchcombe, Poulton, Preston (Cirencester), Preston (Ledbury), Preston upon Stour.

Acton Turville
FOSSETT, W.S., ed. 'Marriages at Acton Turville, 1671 to 1723', *G.P.R.M.* **13**. *P.P.R.S.* **66**, 1908, 69-70.
See also Tormarton.

Alderley
HALE, ROBERT., ed. 'Marriages at Alderley, 1559 to 1812', *G.P.R.M.* **10**. *P.P.R.S.* **43**, 1905, 51-61.

Almondsbury
GREEN, ANGELA. 'An Almondsbury Parish register', *B.G.A.S.Tr.* **78**, 1959, 175-9. Notes on the cover of a lost register.

Alvington
LAMBERT, W.F.A., ed. 'Marriages at Alvington 1698 to 1836', *G.P.R.M.* **14**. *P.P.R.S.* **103**, 1908, 109-14.

Ampney Crucis
JOHNSON, T.C., ed. 'Marriages at Ampney Crucis, 1561 to 1837', *G.P.R.M.* **15**. *P.P.R.S.* **128**, 1909, 103-17.

Arlingham
RAVENHILL, THOMAS HOLMES. 'The parish register of Arlingham', *G.N.Q.* **1**, 1881, 245-8. Includes a few extracts.

Ashchurch
RUSLING, J.W. 'Marriages at Ashchurch, 1555 to 1837', *G.P.R.M.* **14**. *P.P.R.S.* **103**, 1908, 115-42.

Aston sub Edge
B., J. 'Description of an ancient register of the parish of Ashton-sub-Edge, Co. Gloucester, with extracts', *Collectanea topographica et genealogica* **7**, 1841, 279-85. From 1539.
HAMILTON, S.G., ed. 'Marriages at Aston Subedge, 1539 to 1812', *G.P.R.M.* **3**, *P.P.R.S.* **4**, 1898, 59-68.
See also Mickleton.

Aston Somerville
BLOOM, J. HARVEY., ed. 'Marriages at Aston Somerville, 1661 to 1812', *G.P.R.M.* **4**. *P.P.R.S.* **6**, 1896, 5-9.

Avening
EDWARDS, E.W., ed. 'Marriages at Avening, 1557 to 1812', **10**. *P.P.R.S.* **43**, 1905, 1-39.

Badminton
See Great Badminton.

Badsey
See Mickleton.

Batsford
BLOOM, J. HARVEY, ed. 'Marriages at Batsford, 1565 to 1812', *G.P.R.M.* **6**. *P.P.R.S.* **17**, 1900, 1-5.

Berkeley
CRISP, FRED. A., ed. *Parish register of Berkeley, Gloucestershire, 1653-1677*. F. A. Crisp, 1897.
HOLMES, MARGARET. 'Burials of Parliamentarians at Berkeley', *B.G.A.S.Tr.* **72**, 1953, 158-9. 1644-5.

Beverston
SYMONDS, W., ed. 'Marriages at Beverston, 1563 to 1836', *G.P.R.M.* **6**. *P.P.R.S.* **17**, 1900, 7-28.

Bishop's Cleeve
MADGE, SIDNEY J., ed. 'Marriages at Bishop's Cleeve, 1563 to 1812', *G.P.R.M.* **3**. *P.P.R.S.* **4**, 1898, 75-118.

Bitton
CARLYON-BRITTON, W.P., ed. *Registers of Bitton, Baptisms, 1572-1674. Burials, 1572-1668. Marriages, 1571-1674.* Parish Register Society **32**. The Society, 1900.

Bourton on the Water
PRATT, AGATHA, & PRATT, RHODA, eds. 'Marriages at Bourton on the Water, 1654 to 1837', *G.P.R.M.* **17**. *P.P.R.S.* **145**, 1914, 83-109.

Boxwell
BROMEHEAD, J. NOWELL, & FRERE, H.C., eds. 'Marriages at Boxwell and Leighterton, 1572 to 1812', *G.P.R.M.* **13**. *P.P.R.S.* **66**, 1908, 15-21.

Brimpsfield
'Extracts from the Brimpsfield parish registers, 1591-1806', *G.N.Q.* **1**, 1881, 402-5 and 459-61.

Bristol
BAKER, JANE. 'Bristol parishes to 1881', *J.B.A.* **56**, 1989, 23-6. Includes map of parish boundaries, and list of new parishes created 1831-1881, with dates of registers.
HANSOM, J. S., ed. 'Registers of St. Joseph's Chapel, Trenchard Lane (now Street), Bristol, 1707-1808', in *Miscellanea 3*. Catholic Record Society publications **3**. The Society, 1906.

Parish Registers etc. continued

Bristol *continued*
LART, CHARLES EDMUND, ed. *Registers of the French churches of Bristol, Stonehouse, and Plymouth*. Huguenot Society of London publications **20**. The Society, 1912. Bristol baptisms, 1687-1762; marriages, 1688-1744; burials, 1688-1807.

Bristol marriages 1800-1837. Bristol: Bristol & Avon Family History Society, 1980-87:
1. All Saints; St. Mary-le-Pont; Christchurch; St. Nicholas; St. John the Baptist; St. Stephen; St. Werburgh.
2. St. Augustine the Less; St. Georges, Brandon Hill; St. Michael.
3. St. Mary Redcliff; St. Thomas; Temple.
4. St. James.
5. Society of Friends; St. Peter; SS. Philip & Jacob; Holy Trinity; St. Phillips.
6. St. Paul.

There is also a separate volume entitled *Finding Out*, which indexes most of the above.

EMLYN-JONES, S. 'Bristol marriages, 1800-1837', *J.B.A.* **1**, 1975, 13-15. Includes discussion of marriage index, and marriage entries from the parish register of St. Werburgh, 1813-15.
'Gloucestershire marriages in Bristol 1800-1837', *J.G.F.H.S.* **40**, 1989, 30-32; **41**, 1989, 2-22. Strays from various Bristol registers.
HUDLESTON, C. ROY, ed. *The Bristol Cathedral register, 1669-1837*. Bristol: St. Stephen's Bristol Press, 1933.
SABIN, ARTHUR, ed. *The registers of the church of St. Augustine the Less, Bristol, 1577-1700, together with an abstract of the earliest surviving churchwarden's book, 1669-1739*. B.G.A.S. Records branch **3**. Bristol: The Society, 1956. Includes 1714/15 poll book.

Broadwell
LEIGH, Mrs. E.E. 'Marriages at Broadwell, 1605 to 1812' *G.P.R.M.* **14**. *P.P.R.S.* **103**, 1908, 57-69.

Bromesberrow
LLOYD, W. WYNN., ed. 'Marriages at Bromesberrow, 1558 to 1837', *G.P.R.M.* **17**. *P.P.R.S.* **145**, 1914, 1-11.

Brookthorpe
SYMONDS, W., & BLAKE, E.H., eds. 'Marriages at Brookthorpe 1617 to 1812', *G.P.R.M.* **13**, *P.P.R.S.* **66**, 1908, 131-6.

Buckland
BLOOM, J. HARVEY, ed. 'Marriages at Buckland, 1539 to 1839', *G.P.R.M.* **4**. *P.P.R.S.* **6**, 1898, 51-61. Last entry actually 1808.

Bushley
GREENFIELD, BENJ. W. 'Extracts from parish registers (10): Bushley and Thornbury', *G.N.Q.* **3**, 1887, 410-14.

Cam
GRIFFITHS, E.T., ed. 'Marriages at Cam, 1569 to 1812', *G.P.R.M.* **8**. *P.P.R.S.* **29**, 1902, 105-61.

Campden
BARTLEET, S.E. 'Extracts from the Campden register of burials, 1645', *G.N.Q.* **3**, 1887, 213. Of royalist soldiers.

Charlton Kings
ARMITAGE, E.L., ed. *Charlton Kings parish registers*. 2 vols. Cheltenham: Charlton Kings Local History Society, 1983-7. **1**. 1538-1634. **2**. 1634-1700.
MADGE, S.J., ed. 'Marriages at Charlton Kings, 1538 to 1812', *G.P.R.M.* **3**. *P.P.R.S.* **4**, 1897, 119-48.
'Charlton Kings parish register 1635-1700', *C.K.L.H.S.B.* **10**, 1983, 29-35. Brief discussion.
'Charlton Kings persons married in other Gloucestershire parishes: extracts from Phillimore marriage register transcripts', *C.K.L.H.S.B.* **4**, 1980, 31-2.
'Extracts from the Charlton Kings parish register', *G.N.Q.* **1**, 1881, 31-33; **4**, 1890, 331-6. 1538-1811.

Chedworth
HOPE, SACKETT, ed. 'Marriages at Chedworth, 1653 to 1812', *G.P.R.M.* **2**. *P.P.R.S.* **2**, 1897, 133-49.

Cheltenham
MADGE, SIDNEY J., BLAKE, E. H., & RUDGE, S. E., eds. 'Marriages at Cheltenham, 1558 to 1812', *P.P.R.S.* **24**, 1901, 1-118. Includes 20 page introduction.
'Cheltenham parish registers', *G.N.Q.* **8**, 1901, 89-92. Brief description with few extracts.
'Extracts from the Cheltenham parish registers', *G.N.Q.* **1**, 1881, 22, 228-31, 254-6, 295-7, 299-300, and 308-10.
'Longevity of the inhabitants of Cheltenham', *J.G.F.H.S.* **41**, 1989, 24. List of deaths, 1761-1824, of those aged 70+.

Cherington
BROMEHILL, J. NOWILL, & MARRIOTT, C., eds. 'Marriages at Cherington, 1569 to 1812', *G.P.R.M.* **12**. *P.P.R.S.* **63**, 1906, 91-101.

Childswickham
BLOOM, J. HARVEY, ed. 'Marriages at Childswickham 1560-1812, *G.P.R.M.* **4**. *P.P.R.S.* **6**, 1898, 101-14.

Parish Registers etc. continued

Chipping Sodbury
DUMAS, JAMES, ed. 'Marriages at Chipping Sodbury, 1661 to 1812', *G.P.R.M.* **11**. *P.P.R.S* **60**. Phillimore, 1905, 123-41.

Cirencester
MADGE, SIDNEY J. 'Extracts from the register of Cirencester Abbey church', *Genealogist*, N.S. **16**, 1899, 121-5. See also *G.N.Q.* **8**, 1901, 31-2. 16-18th c. Incomplete.
'The registers of Cirencester', *G.N.Q.* **8**, 1901, 31-2. Brief note, including list of 17 registers.

Clifford Chambers
PIPPET, W.A., & BLOOM, J. HARVEY, eds. 'Marriages at Clifford Chambers, 1538 to 1812', *G.P.R.M.* **5**. *P.P.R.S.* **10**, 1899, 133-41. Last entry actually 1808.

Clifton
CAMPBELL, MARY V. *The register of the church of St. Andrew, Clifton (baptisms, burials and marriages 1538-1681)*. Bristol: Bristol Record Society, with Dept. of Extra-Mural Studies, University of Bristol, 1987.

Coaley
PHILLIMORE, W.W., SYMONDS, W., & EVANS, W.J., eds. 'Marriages at Coaley, 1625 to 1812', *G.P.R.M.* **5**. *P.P.R.S.* **10**, 1899, 109-32.
'Coaley parish register extracts', *G.N.Q.* **5**, 1894, 393-7 and 515-8.

Codrington
See Wapley.

Cold Aston
MICHELL, GEORGE B., ed. 'Marriages at Cold Aston, otherwise Aston Blank, 1728 to 1812', in *G.P.R.M.* **17**. *P.P.R.S.* **145**, 1914, 41-6.

Coln Rogers
WOODWARD, G.J., ed. 'Marriages at Coln Rogers 1755 to 1812', *G.P.R.M.* **12**. *P.P.R.S.* **63**, 1906, 149-51.

Didmarton
See Oldbury on the Hill.

Dodington
'Extracts from parish registers (1): Dodington and Doynton', *G.N.Q.* **2**, 1884, 433-6.

Dorsington
BLOOM, J. HARVEY, ed. 'Marriages at Dorsington, 1602 to 1812', *G.P.R.M.* **3**. *P.P.R.S* **4**, 1898, 149-52.

Doynton
See Dodington.

Duntisbourne Abbots
SYMONDS, W., ed. 'Marriages at Duntisbourne Abbots, 1607 to 1837', *G.P.R.M.* **12**. *P.P.R.S.* **63**, 1906, 139-47.

Duntisbourne Rous
TROTTER, A.O., ed. 'Marriages at Duntisbourne Rous, 1549 to 1837', *G.P.R.M.* **17**. *P.P.R.S.* **145**, 1914, 47-56.

Dursley
PHILLIMORE, W.P.W., & Mrs. 'Marriages at Dursley, 1639 to 1812', *G.P.R.M.* **5**. *P.P.R.S.* **10**, 1899, 47-108.

Dymock
GRAY, IRVINE, & GETHYN-JONES, J. E., eds. *The registers of the church of St. Mary, Dymock, 1538-1790*. B.G.A.S. Records Section **4**. Bristol: the Society, 1960.

Dyrham
'Extracts from parish registers (2): Dyrham', *G.N.Q.* **2**, 1884, 536-42 and 592-8.

Eastington
SYMONDS, W., ed. 'Marriages at Eastington, 1558 to 1812', *G.P.R.M.* **13**. *P.P.R.S.* **66**, 1908, 89-122.

Ebrington
BLOOM, J.H., ed. 'Marriages at Ebrington, 1653 to 1812', *G.P.R.M.* **6**. *P.P.R.S.* **17**, 1900, 113-27. See also Mickleton.

Edgeworth
SYMONDS, W., ed. 'Marriages at Edgworth, 1554 to 1812', *G.P.R.M.* **12**. *P.P.R.S.* **63**, 1906, 127-35.

Elkstone
BOUTH, R.H.M., ed. 'Marriages at Elkstone, 1592-1812', *G.P.R.M.* **6**. *P.P.R.S.* **17**, 1900, 103-11.
TONKINSON, THOMAS SILVESTER. *Elkstone: its manors, church and registers*. Cheltenham: Norman Brothers, 1919. Includes many extracts from the parish register, 1593-1797, with list of incumbents *etc*.

Eyford
See Upper Slaughter.

Fairford
CARBONELL, CANON. 'Marriages at Fairford, 1619 to 1837', *G.P.R.M.* **16**. *P.P.R.S.* **143**, 1912, 87-126.

Filton
MACKIE, J.H. 'Marriages at Filton, 1653 to 1812'. *G.P.R.M.* **13**. *P.P.R.S.* **66**, 1908, 53-7.

Forthampton
DOWDESWELL, E.R., ed. 'Marriages at Forthampton, 1678 to 1812', *G.P.R.M.* **1**. *P.P.R.S.* **1**, 1896, 101-11.

Frampton on Severn
'Marriages at Frampton-on-Severn', *G.P.R.M.* **7**. *P.P.R.S.* **24**, 1901, 119-48.

Parish Registers etc. continued

Frocester
SYMONDS, W. 'Marriages at Frocester, 1559 to 1837', *G.P.R.M.* **14**. *P.P.R.S.* **103**, 1908, 1-25. See also *G.N.Q.* **5**, 1893, 369, 404 and 481. 'Frocester marriage register', 1559-1800, *G.N.Q.* **5**, 1894, 369-79, 404-12, and 481-6.

Gloucester
KELSEY, K. 'Looking for a military ancestor?', *J.G.F.H.S.* **37**, 1988, 32. Extracts from Gloucester, Barton Street Chapel and Southgate Street Independent Chapel baptismal registers.
'Extracts from the registers of St. John's, Gloucester', *G.N.Q.* **2**, 1884, 393-8.
'Register book for St. Mary de Lode, A.D. 1656-1659', *Records of Gloucester Cathedral* **3**(1), 1885-97, 35-57.

Great Badminton
TOWER, F., ed. 'Marriages at Great Badminton, 1538 to 1812', *G.P.R.M.* **13**. *P.P.R.S.* **66**, 1908, 23-11.

Great Rissington
PRATT, AGATHA, & PRATT, RHODA, eds. 'Marriages at Great Rissington, 1538 to 1913', *G.P.R.M.* **17**. *P.P.R.S.* **145**, 1914, 57-82.

Guiting Power
BLOOM, J.H., ed. 'Marriages at Guiting Power, 1560 to 1812', *G.P.R.M.* **4**. *P.P.R.S.* **6**, 1896, 125-40.

Hampnett
WIGGIN, WILLIAM. 'The parish registers of Hampnett and Stowell', *G.N.Q.* **1**, 1881, 240-43. Includes a few extracts.
'Marriages in Hampnett, 1737-54', *G.N.Q.* **2**, 1884, **6**, 550-5, and 579-83.

Hanham
FRY, EDW. ALEX., ed. *The register of Hanham and Oldland, Gloucestershire, 1584-1681.* Parish Register Society **63**. Exeter: W. Pollard & Co., 1908.

Hardwicke
BAKER, CATHERINE L. LLOYD, ed. 'Marriages at Hardwicke, 1566 to 1812', *G.P.R.M.* **12**. *P.P.R.S.* **63**, 1906, 71-90.
'Extracts from parish registers (3): Hardwicke', *G.N.Q.* **2**, 1884, 644-5.

Harescombe
HALL, J. MELLAND, ed. 'Marriages at Harescombe 1744 to 1812', *G.P.R.M.* **10**. *P.P.R.S.* **43**, 1905, 63-6.

Hatherop
DOUGLAS, A.W., ed. 'Marriages at Hatherop, 1578 to 1837', *G.P.R.M.* **17**. *P.P.R.S.* **145**, 1914, 31-40.

Hawkesbury
PHILLIMORE, W.P.W., MOSLEY, E.R., & SYMONDS, W., eds. 'Marriages at Hawkesbury, 1603 to 1812', *G.P.R.M.* **5**, *P.P.R.S.* **10**, 1899, 1-46.
'Extracts from the Hawkesbury register', *G.N.Q.* **5**, 1894, 90-92.

Henbury
POYNTON, F.J. 'An account of the early registers at Henbury, Glouc.', *B.G.A.S.Tr.* **12**, 1887-8, 302-22. Includes selected extracts.
POUNTNEY, W., ed. 'Marriages at Henbury, 1544 to 1812', *G.P.R.M.* **16**, *P.P.R.S.* **143**, 1912, 1-71. See also 139-48 for bishops' transcripts.

Hill
VEALE, T., & FUST, JENNER H., eds. 'Marriages at Hill, 1653 to 1812', *G.P.R.M.* **10**. *P.P.R.S.* **43**, 1905, 67-74.

Hinton on the Green
BLOOM, J. HARVEY, ed. 'Marriages at Hinton on the Green, 1735 to 1812', *G.P.R.M.* **4**. *P.P.R.S.* **6**, 1898, 1-3.

Horsley
SYMONDS, W., & DAVIES, W.H. SILVESTER, eds. 'Marriages at Horsley, 1591 to 1811', *G.P.R.M.* **12**. *P.P.R.S.* **63**, 1906, 1-69.

Horton
BEGBIE, OLIVE M., ed. 'Marriages at Horton, 1567 to 1812', *G.P.R.M.* **13**. *P.P.R.S.* **66**, 1908, 1-14.
'Extracts from parish registers, no. IV: Horton', *G.N.Q.* **3**, 1887, 3-5.

Huntley
BLOOD, JOHN N., ed. 'Marriages at Huntley 1583 to 1837', *G.P.R.M.* **16**. *P.P.R.S.* **143**, 1912, 73-86.

Icomb
EVANS, J.T., ed. 'Marriages at Icombe, 1563 to 1812, *G.P.R.M.* **13**. *P.P.R.S.* **66**, 1908, 147-52.

Iron Acton
'Extracts from parish registers (5): Iron Acton', *G.N.Q.* **3**, 1884, 51-5.

Kemerton
MERCIER, J.J., ed. 'Marriages at Kemerton, 1575 to 1716', *G.P.R.M.* **4**. *P.P.R.S.* **6**, 1898, 11-42.

Kempsford
BLACK, W.H. *The registers of Kempsford, Co. Gloucester, 1653-1700.* F.A. Crisp, 1887.
WILLIAMS, ADIN. 'Notes on the parish registers of Kempsford', *G.N.Q.* **5**, 1894, 132-4. General discussion; few extracts.

Parish Registers etc. continued

Kingscote
SYMONDS, W., ed. 'Marriages at Kingscote, 1652 to 1812', *G.P.R.M.* **8**. *P.P.R.S.* **29**, 1902, 97-103.

King's Stanley
'Marriages at King's Stanley, 1573 to 1835', *G.P.R.M.* **1**. *P.P.R.S.* **1**, 1896, 1-55. Actually the last entry is for 1812.

Kingswood
PERKINS, V.R., ed. 'Marriages at Kingswood, 1598 to 1812', *G.P.R.M.* **9**. *P.P.R.S.* **37**, 1903, 105-35.

Leighterton
See Boxwell.

Lemington Parva
BLOOM, J. HARVEY, ed. 'Marriages at Lemington Parva, 1701 to 1812', *G.P.R.M.* **4**. *P.P.R.S.* **6**, 1898, 43-50.

Leonard Stanley
JONES, RICHARD DENISON, ed. 'Marriages at Leonard Stanley, 1570 to 1812', *G.P.R.M.* **2**. *P.P.R.S.* **1**, 1897, 1-23.

Little Rissington
PRATT, AGATHA, & PRATT, RHODA, eds. 'Marriages at Little Rissington, 1550 to 1837', *G.P.R.M.* **17**. *P.P.R.S.* **145**, 1914, 125-35.

Littleton, West
See Tormarton

Long Marston
See Marston Sicca.

Lower Slaughter
'Marriages at Lower Slaughter, 1814 to 1837', *G.P.R.M.* **17**. *P.P.R.S.* **145**, 1914, 111-2.

Maisemore
DIGHTON, CONWAY. 'Maisemore register of baptisms, 1600-1663', *G.N.Q.* **4**, 1890, 497-503 and 524-34. Includes names of clergymen and churchwardens.

DIGHTON, CONWAY. 'Maisemore register of burials, 1538-1599', *G.N.Q.* **4**, 1890, 226-37.

DIGHTON, CONWAY. 'Maisemore register of marriages, 1557-1590', *G.N.Q.* **4**, 1890, 193-6.

DIGHTON, CONWAY, ed. 'Marriages at Maisemore 1557 to 1813', *G.P.R.M.* **14**. *P.P.R.S.* **103**, 1908, 27-41.

Marshfield
[CRISP, FRED. A., ed.] *The parish registers of Marshfield*. F.A. Crisp, 1893. Covers 1558-1693.

Marston Sicca
GARRARD, E.H., ed. 'Marriages at Marston Sicca (otherwise Long Marston)) 1680 to 1812', *G.P.R.M.* **10**. *P.P.R.S.* **43**, 1905, 41-50. Includes a handful of entries from the register bills, 1612 onwards.

Matson
BAZELEY, WILLIAM, ed. 'Marriages at Matson, 1553 to 1812', *G.P.R.M.* **3**. *P.P.R.S.* **4**, 1898, 69-74. Last entry actually 1809.

Mickleton
HAMILTON, S.G., ed. 'Marriages at Mickleton, 1594 to 1812', *G.P.R.M.* **3**, *P.P.R.S.* **4**, 1898, 41-57.

P[HILLIPPS], T[HOMAS]. *Collections for Gloucestershire*. Middle Hill: Medio Montanis, 1861. Extracts from the registers of Mickleton, 1593-1631, Aston Sub Edge, 1566-1718, Ebrington, 1570-1630, Badsey, 1570-1705, and Weston Subedge, 1658-1708.

Minchinhampton
SYMONDS, W., & BRYANS, E.L., & THOMAS, J.A., eds. 'Marriages at Minchinhampton, 1566 to 1812', *G.P.R.M.* **11**. *P.P.R.S.* **60**, 1905, 1-95.

Minsterworth
BARTLETT, CHARLES O., ed. 'Marriages at Minsterworth, 1633 to 1812', *G.P.R.M.* **17**. *P.P.R.S.* **145**, 1914, 13-29.

Mitcheldean
WILKINSON, LEONARD, ed. 'Marriages at Michel Dean, 1680 to 1812', *G.P.R.M.* **9**. *P.P.R.S.* **37**, 1903, 137-54.

Moreton in Marsh
BLOOM, J. HARVEY, ed. 'Marriages at Moreton in Marsh 1672 to 1812', *G.P.R.M.* **5**. *P.P.R.S.* **10**, 1899, 143-56.

Naunton
EALES, E.F., ed. 'Marriages at Naunton, 1545 to 1812', *P.P.R.S.* **128**, 1909, 91-101. Last entry is 1804.

Nether Swell
ROYCE, DAVID, ed. 'Marriages at Nether Swell, 1686 to 1812', *G.P.R.M.* **3**. *P.P.R.S.* **4**, 1898, 1-8.

Newington Bagpath
RUDGE, SELWYN E., & SYMONDS, W., eds. 'Marriages at Newington Bagpath, 1686 to 1812', *G.P.R.M.* **7**. *P.P.R.S.* **24**, 1901, 149-63.

SYMONDS, W., ed. 'Marriages at Newington Bagpath from the bishops' transcripts at Gloucester, additional to those printed in volume 7', *G.P.R.M.* **12**, *P.P.R.S.* **63**, 1906, 111-2.

Parish Registers etc. continued

Nibley, North
See North Nibley.

Nimpsfield
SILVESTER, JAMES, ed. 'Marriages at Nimpsfield, 1679 to 1812', *G.P.R.M.* **1**. *P.P.R.S.* **1**, 1896, 112-31.
SYMONDS, W., ed. 'Marriages at Nimpsfield from the bishops' transcripts at Gloucester, additional to those printed in volume 1', *G.P.R.M.* **12**. *P.P.R.S.* **63**, 1906, 109.

North Nibley
BERKELEY, J.H.C. 'Extracts from the North Nibley parish registers, 1650-1795', *G.N.Q.* **1**, 1881, 364-5.

Oldbury on Severn
SYMONDS, W., ed. 'Marriages at Oldbury on Severn, 1538 to 1733', *G.P.R.M.* **15**. *P.P.R.S.* **128**, 1909, 77-89.

Oldbury on the Hill
SYMONDS, W., ed. 'Marriages at Oldbury on the Hill, and Didmarton, 1568 to 1812', *G.P.R.M.* **11**. *P.P.R.S.* **60**, 1905, 145-54.

Oldland
See Hanham.

Old Sodbury
NASH, CANON. 'Marriages at Old Sodbury, 1684 to 1812', *G.P.R.M.* **9**. *P.P.R.S.* **37**, 1903, 87-104.

Olveston
HAINES, ROBERT J. 'The registers of Olveston, 1560-1812, in the county of Avon, formerly Gloucestershire', *J.B.A.* **6**, 1976, 10-12. General discussion.
HAINES, ROBERT J. 'Some interesting entries in Olveston parish registers', *J.B.A.* **45**, 1986, 37-8.
VERNON, J. E. 'Marriages at Olveston, 1560 to 1812'. *G.P.R.M.* **14**, *P.P.R.S.* **103**, 1908, 71-92. See also Thornbury.

Owlpen
PHILLIMORE, W.P.W., & BENISON, W.B., eds. 'Marriages at Owlpen, 1687 to 1837', *G.P.R.M.* **1**. *P.P.R.S.* **1**, 1896, 57-61.
REDFORD, J. LEMON, ed. 'Marriages at Owlpen, 1837 to 1897', *G.P.R.M.* **2**. *P.P.R.S.* **2**, 1897, 131-2.

Ozleworth
BROMEHEAD, J. NOWILL. 'Marriages at Ozleworth, 1698 to 1812', *G.P.R.M.*, **12**. *P.P.R.S.* **63**, 1906, 103-7.

Painswick
DAVIS, URIAH J., DAVIS, CECIL T., & BADDELEY, W. ST. CLAIR, eds. 'Marriages at Painswick, 1547 to 1812', *G.P.R.M.* **8**. *P.P.R.S.* **29**, 1902, 1-95. To 1757 only. Indicates existence of monumental inscriptions in a 19th c. mss. transcript.
MANSFIELD, GWEN. 'Friends Burial Ground, The Dell Farm, 1658, Painswick, Glos.', *J.G.F.H.S.* **38**, 1988, 11. Loveday family.

Pebworth
WADLEY, THOMAS 'The parish registers of Pebworth: marriages. 1595-1700', *G.N.Q.* **1**, 1881, 274-9. See also 443-5.

Pitchcombe
HALL, J. MELLAND. 'Pitchcombe register of marriages, 1709-42', *G.N.Q.* **3**, 1887, 268-71.

Prestbury
SMITH, H. URLING, ed. 'Marriages at Prestbury 1633 to 1837', *G.P.R.M.* **15**. *P.P.R.S.* **128**, 1909, 129-49.

Preston upon Stour
BLOOM, J. HARVEY, ed. 'Marriages at Preston upon Stour, 1541 to 1812', *G.P.R.M.* **4**. *P.P.R.S.* **6**, 1898, 71-8.

Pucklechurch
'Extracts from parish registers (6): Pucklechurch', *G.N.Q.* **3**, 1887, 67-8.

Quedgeley
BRYANS, E.L., & SYMONDS, W., eds. 'Marriages at Quedgeley, 1559 to 1836', *G.P.R.M.* **1**. *P.P.R.S.* **1**, 1896, 63-78.
'Extracts from the parish registers (7): Quedgeley', *G.N.Q.* **3**, 1887, 87-91, 141-6, and 217-21.

Quinton
BLOOM, J.H., ed. 'Marriages at Quinton, 2 Edward VI [1548] to 1812', *G.P.R.M.* **6**. *P.P.R.S.* **17**, 1900, 69-91.

Rendcombe
KEMPSON, G.A.E., ed. 'Marriages at Rendcombe, 1566 to 1812', *G.P.R.M.* **1**. *P.P.R.S.* **1**, 1896, 79-84. Last entry actually 1810.

Rissington
See under Great, Little and Wyck.

Saintbury
BLOOM, J. HARVEY, ed. 'Marriages at Saintbury, 1585 to 1812', *G.P.R.M.* **4**. *P.P.R.S.* **6**, 1898, 63-70.

Parish Registers etc. continued

Sevenhampton
STORR, WILLIAM R., ed. 'Marriages at Sevenhampton, 1605 to 1837', *G.P.R.M.* **15**. Phillimore, 1909, 119-28.

Sherborne
'Sherborne parish register, 1570-1733', *G.N.Q.* **1**, 1881, 259-61.

Shipton Moyne
SYMONDS, W., ed. 'Marriages at Shipton Moyne, 1587 to 1812', *G.P.R.M.* **9**. *P.P.R.S.* **37**, 1903, 71-85.

Siston
See Syston.

Slaughter
See under Lower and Upper.

Slimbridge
SYMONDS, W., ed. 'Marriages at Slimbridge, 1635 to 1812', *G.P.R.M.* **1**. *P.P.R.S.* **1**, 1896, 133-49.

SYMONDS, W., ed. 'Marriages at Slimbridge: additional entries from 1571 to 1746, from the bishops transcripts at Gloucester', *G.P.R.M.* **11**. *P.P.R.S.* **60**, 1905, 115-22.

Snowshill
'Marriages at Snowshill, 1593 to 1603', *G.P.R.M.* **4**. *P.P.R.S.* **6**, 1898, 91.

Southrop
SQUIRE, MRS., ed. 'Marriages at Southrop, 1656 to 1837', *G.P.R.M.* **13**. *P.P.R.S.* **66**, 1908, 137-46.

Standish
SYMONDS, W., ed. 'Marriages at Standish, 1559 to 1812', *G.P.R.M.* **6**. *P.P.R.S.* **17**, 1900, 29-68.

Stanton
BLOOM, J. HARVEY, ed. 'Marriages at Stanton, 1572 to 1812', *G.P.R.M.* **4**. *P.P.R.S.* **6**, 1898, 79-90.

Stinchcombe
LYNCH-BLOSSE, R.C., ed. 'Marriages at Stinchcombe, 1583 to 1812', *G.P.R.M.* **6**. *P.P.R.S.* **17**, 1900, 129-48. Supersedes edition in vol. **2**, which excludes entries for 1754-84, then missing.

Stone
CRIPPS, C., & SYMONDS, W., eds. 'Marriages at Stone, 1594 to 1812', *G.P.R.M.* **3**. *P.P.R.S.* **4**, 1898, 9-40.

Stonehouse
JONES, RICHARD DENISON, ed. 'Marriages at Stonehouse, 1558 to 1812', *G.P.R.M.* **2**. *P.P.R.S.* **2**, 1897, 25-74.

'Memoranda in the Stonehouse register', *G.N.Q.* **7**, 1890, 8-11. Mainly concerning vicars.

Stowell
See Hampnett.

Sudeley
See Winchcombe.

Swell, Nether
See Nether Swell.

Swindon
M[ADGE], S.J., 'Extracts from Swindon parish registers, 1606-1838', *G.N.Q.* **9**, 1902, 71-80.

MADGE, SIDNEY, ed. 'Marriages at Swindon, 1638 to 1837', *G.P.R.M.* **1**. *P.P.R.S.* **1**, 1896, 85-100.

MADGE, S.J. 'Swindon surnames, 1606-1838', *G.N.Q.* **9**, 1902, 139-60. Effectively an index to some volumes of the parish register.

Syde
SYMONDS, W., ed. 'Marriages at Syde, 1686 to 1812', *G.P.R.M.* **12**. *P.P.R.S.* **63**, 1906, 137-8.

Syston
McCALL, H.B., ed. *The parish register of Syston or Siston, in the county of Gloucester, from 1576-1641*. Nailsworth: the editor, 1901.

'Extracts from parish registers, no. VIII: Syston', *G.N.Q.* **3**, 1887, 236-8.

Temple Guiting
BLOOM, J.H., ed. 'Marriages at Temple Guiting, 1676 to 1752', *G.P.R.M.* **4**. *P.P.R.S.* **6**, 1898, 83-7. The last marriage recorded is actually 1771.

Tetbury
KITCAT, A., ed. 'Marriages at Tetbury, 1631 to 1812', *G.P.R.M.* **10**. *P.P.R.S.* **43**, 1905, 75-153.

WRIGLEY, E.A. 'Clandestine marriage in Tetbury in the late 17th century', *Local population studies* **10**, 1973, 15-21. Discussion of some reasons for the failure to record marriages in parish registers.

'Extracts from the Tetbury parish registers: burials, 1658-1811', *G.N.Q.* **1**, 1881, 323-5.

Parish Registers etc. continued

Thornbury
SYMONDS, W., & COMMELINE, MISS. 'Marriages at Thornbury 1550 to 1812', *G.P.R.M.* **15**. *P.P.R.S.* **128**, 1909, 1-76.

ROE, E. A. 'Thornbury marriages missing from Phillimore's Glouc., vol. no. **15**', *Genealogists magazine* **13**, 1959-61, 246-50. Covers 1663-70, 1679-83, and 1718-28.

'Extracts from parish registers, no. IX: Thornbury and Olveston', *G.N.Q.* **3**, 1887, 256-7.
See also Bushley.

Tidenham
KEYTE, F.H., & M., eds. *Tidenham parish register*. Chepstow Society pamphlet series **7** and **10**. Chepstow: the Society, 1960-71.

Tirley
RUSLING, J.W., ed. 'Marriages at Tirley, 1655 to 1812', *G.P.R.M.* **14**. *P.P.R.S.* **103**, 1903, 43-56.

Todenham
BLOOM, J. HARVEY, ed. 'Marriages at Todenham, 1721 to 1812', *G.P.R.M.* **4**. *P.P.R.S.* **6**, 1898, 147-53.

Tormarton
SYMONDS, W., ed. 'Marriages at Tormarton with West Littleton, 1600 to 1812; including Acton Turville, 1754 to 1812', *G.P.R.M.* **13**. *P.P.R.S.* **66**, 1908, 71-87.

Tortworth
MOSLEY, E.R., ed. 'Marriages at Tortworth, 1620 to 1812', *G.P.R.M.* **12**. *P.P.R.S.* **63**, 1906, 113-25.

Tredington
MACLEAN, JOHN. 'The plague at Tredington, 1610-11', *G.N.Q.* **2**, 1884, 71-3. Extracts from the parish register.

Turkdean
BISCOE, FREDERICK. 'Turkdean parish registers etc.', *G.N.Q.* **1**, 1881, 284-5. Includes a few extracts.

GREENING, G.H.B., ed. 'Marriages at Turkdean, 1572 to 1837', *G.P.R.M.* **14**. *P.P.R.S.* **103**, 1908, 140-56.

TUDOR, J.L. 'The registers of Turkdean parish', *G.N.Q.* **2**, 1884, 199-200, 257-9, and 449-52.

Twining
DOWDESWELL, E.R., ed. 'Marriages at Twining, 1674 to 1812', *G.P.R.M.* **13**. *P.P.R.S.* **66**, 1908, 35-51.

Uley
BENISON, W.B. ed. 'Marriages at Uley, 1668 to 1812, *G.P.R.M.* **2**, *P.P.R.S.* **2**, 1897, 89-129.
'Notes about Uley', *G.N.Q.* **5**, 1894, 6-12 and 64-7. Primarily parish register extracts.

Upper Slaughter
PRATT, AGATHA & PRATT, RHODA, eds. 'Marriages at Upper Slaughter with Eyford 1538 to 1837', *G.P.R.M.* **17**. *P.P.R.S.* **145**, 1914, 113-24.

Wapley
'Gloucestershire strays', *J.G.F.H.S.* **5**, 1980, 14. Extracts from registers of Wapley and Codrington, relating to other Gloucestershire parishes.

Westbury on Trym
WILKINS, H.J., ed. *The church register (A.D. 1559-1713) of the ancient parish of Westbury-upon-Trym*. Westbury and Bristol records 3. Bristol: J.W. Arrowsmith, 1912.

Westcote
LAMBERT, W.F.A. 'Marriages at Westcote, 1630 to 1812', *G.P.R.M.* **14**. *P.P.R.S.* **103**, 1908, 143-8.

West Littleton
See Tormarton.

Weston Birt
SYMONDS, W., ed. 'Marriages at Weston Birt, 1596 to 1812', *G.P.R.M.* **6**. *P.P.R.S.* **17**, 1900, 149-55.

Weston sub Edge
BLOOM, J. HARVEY, ed. 'Marriages at Weston Subedge, 1612 to 1812', *G.P.R.M.* **4**. *P.P.R.S.* **6**, 1898, 115-24.
See also Mickleton.

Whaddon
H. 'Transcript of Whaddon parish register, 1674-1711', *G.N.Q.* **4**, 1890, 375-82.

SYMONDS, W., & BLAKE, E.H., eds. 'Marriages at Whaddon, 1620 to 1812', *G.P.R.M.* **13**. *P.P.R.S.* **66**, 1908, 123-30.

Wickwar
MALDEN, HENRY C., ed. 'Marriages at Wickwar, 1689 to 1812', *G.P.R.M.* **11**. *P.P.R.S.* **60**, 1905, 97-114.

Willersey
BARTLETT, F., & BLOOM, J.H., eds. 'Marriages at Willersey, 1723 to 1812', *G.P.R.M.* **6**. *P.P.R.S.* **17**, 1900, 93-101.

Parish Registers etc. continued

Winchcombe
TAYLOR, JOHN. 'Winchcombe parish registers', *Gloucester diocesan magazine* **2**, 1907, 32-5 and 57-9. General discussion.
WEBB, T.C., ed. 'Marriages at Winchcombe, 1539 to 1812', *G.P.R.M.* **9**. *P.P.R.S.* **37**, 1903, 1-70.
'Parish registers of Winchcombe and Sudeley', *G.N.Q.* **1**, 1881, 113-4 and 140. List of register books; almost no extracts.

Windrush
'Windrush parish registers 1586-1732', *G.N.Q.* **1**, 1881, 265-6. Brief description of the registers.

Winstone
TROTTER, A., ed. 'Marriages at Winstone, 1540 to 1837', *G.P.R.M.* **16**. *P.P.R.S.* **143**, 1912, 127-38.

Woodchester
GETHEN, M. A., & HOUGH, L., eds. *Liber baptismi et confirmat: baptisms and confirmations at Woodchester, 1846-1859.* [ ]: Gloucestershire & North Avon Catholic History Society, 1989.

Woolaston
LAMBERT, W.F.A., ed. 'Marriages at Woolaston, 1696 to 1837', *G.P.R.M.* **14**. *P.P.R.S.* **103**, 1908, 93-107.

Wormington
BLOOM, J. HARVEY, ed. 'Marriages at Wormington, 1719 to 1812', *G.P.R.M.* **4**. *P.P.R.S.* **6**, 1898, 99-100.

Wyck Risington
KEMPTHORNE, H., ed. 'Marriages at Wyck Risington, 1605 to 1838', *G.P.R.M.* **13**. *P.P.R.S.* **66**, 1908, 59-67.

9. PROBATE RECORDS AND INQUISITIONS POST MORTEM

A. GENERAL

Probate records – wills, inventories, administration bonds *etc.* – are invaluable sources of genealogical information. For Gloucestershire, most wills were proved in the Consistory courts of the bishops of Gloucester and Bristol. Records from these and other courts are listed in:
PHILLIMORE, W.P.W., & DUNCAN, LELAND L., eds. *A calendar of wills proved in the Consistory Court of the Bishop of Gloucester.* Index Library **12** and **34**. British Record Society, 1895-1907. **1**. 1541-1650, with an appendix of dispersed wills and wills proved in the peculiar courts of Bibury and Bishops Cleeve. **2**. 1660-1800, ed. Edw. Alexander Fry & W.P.W. Phillimore.
FRY, EDWARD ALEXANDER, ed. *A calendar of wills proved in the Consistory Court (city and deanery of Bristol) of the Bishop of Bristol, 1572-1792, and also a calendar of wills in the Great Orphan Books preserved in the Council House, Bristol, 1379-1674.* Index Library **17**. British Record Society, 1897.
GEORGE, E.S. *Guide to the probate inventories of the Bristol deanery of the Diocese of Bristol (1542-1804).* Bristol: B.G.A.S. and Bristol Record Society, 1988.
Prior to 1541, Gloucestershire was an Archdeaconry within the Diocese of Worcester. A very few Gloucestershire wills are therefore listed in:
FRY, EDW. ALEX., ed. *Calendar of wills and administrations in the Consistory Court of the Bishop of Worcester, 1451-1600...* Index Library **31**. British Record Society, 1910. Also issued by the Worcestershire Historical Society.
A number of other courts also exercised probate jurisdiction in Bristol and Gloucestershire. See:
DICKINSON, MICHAEL G. *Wills proved in Gloucestershire peculiar courts.* Local history pamphlet **2**. Gloucester: City Libraries, 1960. For Bibury, Bishop's Cleeve and Withington; supplements Phillimore & Duncan's calendar noted above.
MAYO, C.H. 'Calendar of wills in the archives of the Dean and Chapter of the Cathedral of Bristol', *Notes & queries for Somerset & Dorset* **13**, 1913, 153-61. Somerset, Dorset and Gloucestershire.
'Gloucestershire wills at Somerset House 1418-1543', *G.N.Q.* **8**, 1901, 30. Brief list, 1418-1583, of Prerogative Court of Canterbury wills.

Probate Records Etc.: General continued

Despite the title, a few interregnum administrations for Gloucestershire, as well as Cornwall and Somerset, are listed in:

FRY, G.S. 'Dorset administrations', *Notes & queries for Somerset & Dorset* **2**, 1891, 14-16, 52-5, 87-9, 132-5, 189-92, 226-9, 270-2 and 295-8; **3**, 1893, 12-15, 49-52, 83, 93-6, 146-8, 165-9, 213-6, 261-4 and 316-9; **4**, 1895, 25-7, 58-61, 103-5, 146-9, 213-5, 250-3, 306-9 and 361-4; **5**, 1897, 23-6, 65-9, 116-21, 158-62, 206-10, 257-62, 301-8, and 339-45; **6**, 1899, 26-31, 57-61, 110-14, 154-8, 210-12, 247-9, 234-7, and 356-8.

GENEALOGIST. 'A list of Gloucestershire wills', *G.N.Q.* **2**, 1884, 348-9. From Coleman's *Catalogue of 1000 wills.* 1883.

Many wills and inventories have been published in part or fully. Brief abstracts are provided in: 'Gloucestershire wills', *G.N.Q.* **5**, 1894, 45-7, 98-102, 147-56, 271-2, 331-2, 365-8, 416-8 and 561-6.; **6**, 1896, 72-4.

B. BY PLACE

A number of probate record collections relating to specific places are available:

Bristol

McGRATH, PATRICK. *Bristol wills.* 2 vols. Bristol: University of Bristol Dept. of Extra-Mural Studies, 1975-8. **1**. 1546-1593. **2**. 1597-1598.

WADLEY, T.P. *Notes or abstracts of the wills contained in the volume entitled the Great Orphan Book and Book of Wills, in the Council House at Bristol.* Bristol: C.T. Jefferies & Sons for B.G.A.S., 1886. 1381-1595.

McGRATH, PATRICK V. 'The wills of Bristol merchants in the Great Orphan Books', *B.G.A.S.Tr.* **68**, 1949, 91-109. General discussion.

SABIN, ARTHUR. 'Bristol wills and documents', *B.G.A.S.Tr.* **64**, 1943, 118-47. Includes 10 wills of 1559 from the Consistory Court, with other court papers.

BURGESS, CLIVE. 'By quick and by dead: wills and pious provision in late medieval Bristol', *English historical review* **102**, 1987, 837-58.

Charlton Kings

'Charlton Kings wills, 1547-1558: some interim conclusions', *C.K.L.H.S.B.* **6**, 1981, 25-30.

GREET, M.J. 'Early wills from Charlton Kings', *C.K.L.H.S.B.* **4**, 1980, 5-16. Includes notes on 16th c. wills, and on curates.

By Place continued

Cirencester

BISHOP, G.L., ed. *Wills from Cirencester and district, 1541-1548.* Cirencester: the editor, 1987.

Clifton

MOORE, JOHN S., ed. *Clifton and Westbury probate inventories 1609-1761.* Bristol: Avon Local History Association, 1981.

Forest of Dean

OWEN, BARBARA. 'Forest wills and testaments', *New regard* **6**, 1990, 26-9. Brief notes.

Frampton Cotterell

MOORE, JOHN S., ed. *The goods and chattels of our forefathers: Frampton Cotterell and district probate inventories, 1539-1804.* Frampton Cotterell and district historical studies **1**. Phillimore, 1976.

Gloucester

AUSTIN, ROLAND. 'Gloucester wills', *B.G.A.S.Tr.* **60**, 1938, 354-5. Brief list of wills in Stevenson's *Calendar of the records of the Corporation of Gloucester.*

Mangotsfield

JONES, PERIS. 'Probate inventories for Mangotsfield parish 1611-1670', *J.B.A.* **36**, 1984, 23-8. List.

WILSON, JOHN. 'Mangotsfield wills, [1593-1671]', *J.B.A.* **2**, 1975, 8; **3**, 1976, 24; and **7**, 1977, 22. List of wills proved in the Bristol diocesan Consistory Court.

Westbury

See Clifton.

C. BY FAMILY

Many individual wills and inventories have been separately published, and are listed below:

Arnolde

HALL, J. MELLAND. 'The will of John Arnolde, rector of St Michaels, Gloucester, 1450', *G.N.Q.* **2**, 1884, 532-3.

Arundel

HEANE, W.C. 'The Arundel family', *G.N.Q.* **5**, 1894, 110-11. 3 wills.

See also Merryweather.

Bathe

ABHBH. 'Two early English wills, 1420 and 1438', *G.N.Q.* **3**, 1887, 317-8. Wills of John Bathe and Richard Dixton.

Biddill

See Sawnders.

Probate Records etc.: By Family continued

Birche
'Gloucestershire wills', *G.N.Q.* **10**, 1914, 17-21. Wills of George Birche of Uley, 1610, Langley family 15th c., and John Gale of Little Sodbury, 1588.

Birt
NIBLETT, ARTHUR. 'The will of Samuel Birt, of Haresfield, with inventory', *G.N.Q.* **4**, 1890, 467-8.

Blake
See Williams.

Broadway
WADLEY, THOMAS. 'The Broadway family', *G.N.Q.* **1**, 1881, 123-5. Includes will of Edmund Bradwey, 1493.

Browning
See Merryweather.

Burcombe
'Burcombe beneficiaries', *J.G.F.H.S.* **41**, 1989, 29; **44**, 1990, 25. Extracts from Burcombe family wills, 16-17th c.

Butler
H., J.M. 'Two old Gloucestershire wills, 1595', *G.N.Q.* **3**, 1887, 677-8. Robert Butler and Henry Watkins.

Camber
HALL, J. MELLAND. 'The will of John Camber, 1496', *G.N.Q.* **2**, 1894, 444-6.

Capel
'The will of the Rev. Richard Capel, M.A.', *G.N.Q.* **2**, 1884, 638-42. 1656.

Clutterbuck
C., R.H. 'Will of Robert Clutterbuck, 1563', *G.N.Q.* **5**, 1894, 329-30.
'Will of Richard Clutterbuck of Eastington, 1583', *G.N.Q.* **5**, 1894, 229-30.

Creswicke
'Will of Alderman Francis Creswicke', *Notes &d queries for Somerset & Dorset* **14**, 1915, 14-15. Of Bristol, 1646.

Daston
WADLEY, THOMAS 'The will of John Daston of Dumbleton 1530', *G.N.Q.* **3**, 1887, 668-9.

Daunsey
See Merryweather.

Deen
HALL, J. MELLARD. 'Shipton Oliffe: will of Giles Deen, A.D. 1634', *G.N.Q.* **4**, 1890, 132-4.

Diston
AUSTIN, ROLAND. 'The inventory of the goods of Oliver Diston, rector of Dumbleton, Gloucestershire, 1615', *B.G.A.S.Tr.* **46**, 1924, 187-93.

Dixton
FULLER, E.A. 'The will of Richard Dixton esq.', *B.G.A.S.Tr.* **11**, 1886-7, 155-60. 1438.
See also Bathe.

Elyce
WADLEY, THOMAS 'Notes on the wills of two Wotton under Edge worthies', *G.N.Q.* **2**, 1884, 19-20. Robert Elyce, 1508, and Robert Looge, 1508.

French
See Williams.

Gale
See Birche.

Giffard
HALL, J. MELLAND. 'The will of Godfrey Giffard, Bishop of Worcester, A.D. 1301', *B.G.A.S.Tr.* **20**, 1895-7, 139-54.

Hart
GREENFIELD, BENJ. 'Abstract of the will of Richard Hart, last Prior of Lanthony', *G.N.Q.* **2**, 1884, 305. 1545.
See also Williams.

Harvey
HARVEY, WM. M. 'Will of the Rev. John Harvey, of Iron Acton 1693 *etc.*', *G.N.Q.* **3**, 1887, 503-5.

Heavens
[Will of Arthur Heavens, 1849], *J.G.F.H.S.* **26**, 1985, 5-6.

Hodges
WADLEY, THOMAS. 'The will of Laurence Hodges, 1514', *G.N.Q.* **1**, 1881, 143-4.

Horton
'Notes of old Gloucestershire wills', *G.N.Q.* **1**, 1881, 97-8. Wills of William Horton, 1537, and John Tomes, 1537.

Huntington
AUSTIN, ROLAND. 'The will of Robert Huntington, vicar of Leigh, 1648-1664', *B.G.A.S.Tr.* **58**, 1936, 243-56.

Hutchens
See Payne.

Langley
See Birche.

Probate Records etc.: By Family continued

Looge
See Elyce.

Lyne
LYNE, ROBT. EDWIN. 'The Lyne family', *G.N.Q.* **2**, 1884, 89-91. List of wills.

Lynett
GREET, M.J. 'A dispute over the will of Alice Lynett, 1551-1553', *C.K.L.H.S.B.* **5**, 1981, 7-11.

Marshall
MARSHALL, GEORGE W. 'A priest's will in 1528', *G.N.Q.* **1**, 1881, 105-7. Will of Thomas Marshall.

Merryweather
'Gloucestershire wills', *G.N.Q.* **7**, 1900, 95-6. Francis Merryweather of Uley, 1660; Mary Arundell of Stroud, 1660; Christopher Daunsey of Uley, 1604; Thomas Browning of Gloucester, 1608.

Michell
HALL, J. MELLAND. 'Harescombe: the will of James Michell', *G.N.Q.* **4**, 1890, 164-7.

Miles
'An ancient inventory', *G.N.Q.* **6**, 1896, 33-6. Thomas Miles, *c.*16-17th c.

Morgan
See Payne.

Morton
FINBERG, H.P.R. 'Sir Robert Morton's will', in his *Gloucestershire studies*. Leicester: Leicester University Press, 1957, 121-2.
FULLER, E.A. 'Cirencester documents', *B.G.A.S.Tr.* **20**, 1895-96, 114-26. Includes will of Sir Robert Morton, 1493.

Myll
HALL, J. MELLAND. 'The will of Thomas Myll, of Harescombe, A.D. 1509', *G.N.Q.* **3**, 1887, 626.

Overbury
'Additional notes on the family of Overbury', *Genealogist* **1**, 1877, 394. Will of Thomas Overbury of Aston-sub-Edge, 1545.

Payne
HALL, J. MELLAND. 'Four Brockthorpe wills', *G.N.Q.* **4**, 1890, 466-7. Wills of Robert Payne, George Morgan and Arthur Sowle, 1598, and Thomas Smythe alias Hutchens, 1611.

Poulton
DUNCAN, LELAND L. 'The family of Poulton', *G.N.Q.* **6**, 1896, 1-3, and 69-72. Wills.

Prowde
WADLEY, THOMAS 'Two Bristol wills, A.D. 1500-1502', *G.N.Q.* **3**, 1887, 534. Thomas Prowde and John Walter.

Pynke
PINK, W.D. 'Will of John Pynke, of Bristol, 1494', *G.N.Q.* **4**, 1890, 325-6.

See also 389-90.

Redcle
HALL, J. MELLAND. 'The will of John Redcle, of Pychyncumbe, 1537', *G.N.Q.* **2**, 1884, 573. Pitchcombe.

Rodway
WADLEY, THOMAS. 'The Rodway family of Rodborough', *G.N.Q.* **3**, 1887, 260-61. 16th c. wills.

Rogers
'Extract from the will of John Rogers, 1695', *G.N.Q.* **1**, 1881, 331-2.

Rutter
WADLEY, THOMAS. 'Will of Richard Rutter, of Alderton, 1545', *G.N.Q.* **4**, 1890, 182-3. See also 33-4.

Sawnders
'Some early Gloucestershire wills', *G.N.Q.* **10**, 1913, 44. Thomas Sawnders alias Biddill, 1487.

Selk
MACLEAN, SIR JOHN. 'The will of William Selk, vicar of All Saints, Bristol, 1270', *B.G.A.S.Tr.* **15**, 1890-1, 310-315.

Shipton
PARTRIDGE, J.B. 'A yeoman's house in the eighteenth century', *Gloucestershire countryside* **3**(3), 1938, 334-5. Inventory of Abraham Shipton, 1743.

Smith
GRAY, IRVINE. 'Smith of Nibley's will', *B.G.A.S.Tr.* **78**, 1959, 129-36. John Smith, 1640/41.

Smythe
See Payne.

Somers
P[HILLIMORE], W.P.W. 'Somers family', *G.N.Q.* **5**, 1894, 53. Will of Lawrence Somers, 1620.

Probate Records etc.: By Family continued

Sowle
See Payne.

Stafford
G., B.W. 'Will of John Stafford of Marlwood, esq., 1596', *Topographer & genealogist* **1**, 1846, 142-4.

Stradlynge
J., D. 'John Stradlynge, of Stanley St Leonards, 1558', *G.N.Q.* **4**, 1890, 395. Note on his will.

Sturmy
HICKS, F.W. POTTO. 'Robert Sturmy of Bristol', *B.G.A.S.Tr.* **60**, 1938, 169-79. Includes will, 1457.

Tomes
See Horton.

Wakeman
See Williams.

Ware
See Williams.

Walter
See Prowde.

Watkins
See Butler.

Watts
'A sad little will', *History of Tetbury Society journal* **19**, 1988, 9-12. Margaret Watts, 1612.

Wayte
'Gloucestershire wills', *G.N.Q.* **7**, 1900, 177-80 and 190; **8**, 1901, 18. Wayte family wills, 16-18th c.

White
WAY, LEWIS J. UPTON. 'An inventory of the goods of John White of Drystowe taken in 1559', *B.G.A.S.Tr.* **43**, 1921, 267-78.

Whittington
ALLEN, W. TAPNELL. 'The will of William Whittington, of St. Briavels, gent., 1625', *B.G.A.S.Tr.* **10**, 1885-6, 304-12.

Williams
BASKERVILLE, G. 'Some ecclesiastical wills', *B.G.A.S.Tr.* **52**, 1930, 281-93. Includes wills of Morgan Williams, 1543, Richard Hart, 1545, Thomas Ware, 1546, William French, 1548, John Wakeman, 1549, and John Blake, 1552.

Wytloff
'Will of John Wytloff, of Ladyswill, 1494', *G.N.Q.* **2**, 1884, 403-4. Devon, made at Bristol.

D. INQUISITIONS POST MORTEM

Inquisitions post mortem are invaluable sources of genealogical information for the medieval period, and are particularly useful in tracing the descent of manors. They were taken on the deaths of tenants in chief, and recorded lands held, with the names of heirs. For Gloucestershire, abstracts are printed in:

Abstracts of Gloucestershire inquisitiones post mortem returned into the Court of Chancery. Index Library **9**, **13**, **21**, **30**, **40** and **47**. British Record Society, 1893-1914. **1**. Charles I, 1625-1636, ed. W.P.W. Phillimore & George S. Fry; **2**. Charles I, 1637-1645; **3**. Miscellaneous series, 1-18 Charles I, 1625-1642, ed., Edw. Alexander Fry; **4**. 20 Henry III to 29 Edward I, 1236-1300, ed. Sidney J. Madge; **5**. 30 Edward I to 32 Edward III, 1302-1358, ed., Edward Alexander Fry; **6**. 33 Edward III to 14 Henry IV, 1359-1413, ed., Ethel Stokes.

See also

'Early chancery inquisitions, 1236-1272', *G.N.Q.* **8**, 1901, 46-9. List.

PHILLIMORE, W.P.W. 'Gloucestershire inquisitones post mortem', *G.N.Q.* **3**, 1887, 346-8. Select list, 1546-1641.

The inquisition taken on the death of Robert Waleraund is printed in:

'Siston manor, 1273', *G.N.Q.* **8**, 1901, 49-50.

10. MONUMENTAL INSCRIPTIONS

A. GENERAL

Monumental inscriptions are an important source of genealogical information. Many have been transcribed; lists of transcriptions are provided by:
RAWES, JULIAN. *Catalogue of memorial lists of Gloucestershire*. [ ]: G.F.H.S., 1988.
AUSTIN, ROLAND. 'Churchyard inscriptions: list of transcriptions', *Notes & queries*, series **11**(7), 1913, 110-11.
A number of attempts have been made to record Gloucestershire inscriptions since 1791. A useful discussion of these various projects is provided by:
'Gloucestershire's memorial inscriptions', *J.G.F.H.S.* **44**, 1990, 27-8.
For the records of Bristol cemeteries, see:
BRISTOL RECORD OFFICE. *Records of cemeteries and private burial grounds*. Information leaflet **6**. Bristol: the Office, 1989.
Brief description of monuments in many Gloucestershire churches are provided by:
ROBINSON, W.J. *West country churches*. 4 vols. Bristol: Bristol Times & Mirror, 1914-16. This also covers East Somerset and Wiltshire.
The standard account of monumental effigies is:
ROPER, IDA M. *The monumental effigies of Gloucestershire and Bristol*. Gloucester: Henry Osborne, 1931.
There are also a number of briefer works:
BAGNALL-OAKLEY, MARY ELLEN. 'List of monumental effigies in Bristol and Gloucestershire', *B.G.A.S.Tr.* **25**, 1902, 148-81.
BAGNALL-OAKLEY, MARY ELLEN. 'On some sculptured effigies of ecclesiastics in Gloucestershire', *B.G.A.S.Tr.* **9**, 1884-5, 51-71.
FRYER, ALFRED C. 'Monumental effigies made by Bristol craftsmen [1240-1550]', *Archaeologia* **74**, 1925, 1-72. In Bristol, Gloucestershire, Somerset, Wales and various other places.
HARTSHORNE, ALBERT. 'Observations upon certain monumental effigies in the West of England, particularly in the neighbourhood of Cheltenham', *B.G.A.S.Tr.* **4**, 1879-80, 231-47.
'On certain rare monumental effigies', *B.G.A.S.Tr.* **25**, 1902, 94.
For monumental brasses, see:
DAVIS, CECIL T. *The monumental brasses of Gloucestershire*. Bath: Kingsmead Reprints, 1969. Originally published Phillimore, 1899.
DAVIS, CECIL T. 'The monumental brasses of Gloucestershire', *Archaeological journal* **48**, 1891, 19-28.
FRANKS, A.W. '[Notes on the monumental brasses of Gloucestershire]', *Proceedings of the Society of Antiquaries of London*, series **2**(7), 1878, 409-13. Brief note.

General continued

'Monumental brasses in Gloucestershire', *G.N.Q.* **1**, 1881, 137-9 and 142-3. Brief note.
For inscriptions relating to Gloucestershire in other places, see:
GENEALOGIST. 'Monumental inscriptions from Jamaica and Barbados', *G.N.Q.* **2**, 1884, 295-9. Relating to Gloucestershire.
'Monumental inscriptions from other counties', *G.N.Q.* **4**, 1890, 534-9.

B. BY PLACE

Almondsbury
ABHBA. 'Almondsbury church: monumental inscriptions', *G.N.Q.* **4**, 1890, 4-11.

Badgeworth
RAWES, J.A. 'Badgeworth (Holy Trinity) Church', *J.G.F.H.S.* **27**, 1985, 12-13. Five nineteenth century inscriptions.

Beckington
PARRY, H. 'Notes on brasses in churches (illustrated) at Beckington, Cirencester and St. Mary Redcliffe, Bristol', *Somerset Archaeological & National History Society. Proceedings of the Bath & District branch*, 1919-23, 117-20.

Berkeley
COOKE, JAMES HERBERT. 'On the ancient inscriptions in the chapel at Berkeley Castle with some account of John Trevisa', *B.G.A.S.Tr.* **1**, 1876, 138-46.

Bisley
SWALE, A. *All Saints, Bisley: a guide to identifiable graves and memorials in the churchyard and church*. Bisley: the author, 1986.

Brimscombe
ABHBA. 'Brimscombe Church: momumental inscriptions', *G.N.Q.* **4**, 1890, 459-61.
'Index to monumental inscriptions: Brimscombe, Cainscross, Edge, Nailsworth, Oakridge, Sheepscombe and Slade', *G.N.Q.* **1**, 1881, 214-5.

Bristol
ABHBA. 'Christ Church Bristol: monumental inscriptions', *G.N.Q.* **4**, 1890, 656-61.
ABHBA. 'St George's, Brandon Hill, Bristol: monumental inscriptions', *G.N.Q.* **4**, 1890, 584-5.
ABHBA. 'St. Nicholas Church, Bristol: monumental inscriptions', *G.N.Q.* **4**, 1890, 240-6.

Monumental Inscriptions: By Place continued

Bristol *continued*

BARKER, W.R. 'On the later monuments in the mayor's chapel', *B.G.A.S.Tr.* **15**, 1890-91, 76-88.

OWEN, LES. 'Arno's Vale cemetery', *J.B.A.* **59**, 1990, 29-33. Private burial in Bristol; article includes note on the cemetery's records.

ROPER, IDA M. *The history and memorials of St. Mark's Church, Bristol, which is now the Lord Mayor's Chapel (formerly called the Church of the Gaunts)*. Bristol: W.C. Hemmons, 1913. Includes brief notes on some memorials.

WADE, EDWARD FRY. 'St. Werburgh's Church, Bristol: monumental inscriptions', *G.N.Q.* **4**, 1890, 558-63.

'Effigies of Bristol', *B.G.A.S.Tr.* **26**, 1903, 215-87; **27**, 1904, 51-116.

'Index to monumental inscriptions: St. George's, Brandon Hill, Bristol', *G.N.Q.* **2**, 1884, 137-8.

See also Beckington, Redland.

Bristol Deanery

ROPER, IDA M. 'Monumental effigies: rural deanery of Bristol', *B.G.A.S.Tr.* **34**, 1911, 126-60.

Brockworth

D., C.T. 'Brockworth church: monumental inscriptions', *G.N.Q.* **4**, 1890, 577-9.

'Index to monumental inscriptions, Brockworth', *G.N.Q.* **1**, 1881, 387-8.

Cainscross

ABHBA. 'Cainscross church: monumental inscriptions', *G.N.Q.* **4**, 1890, 403-5.

See also Brimscombe.

Cerney, North

See North Cerney.

Chalford

'Index to monumental inscriptions *etc.*, Chalford', *G.N.Q.* **1**, 1881, 135-7, and **4**, 1890, 404-5. Includes transcripts of nine inscriptions.

Charlton Kings

BLACKER, BEAVER H. *Monumental inscriptions in the parish church of Charlton Kings, with extracts from the parish registers, and some churchyard inscriptions*. Privately printed, 1876.

FLETCHER, SIMON. 'Memorials in St. Mary's Church, Charlton Kings', *C.K.L.H.S.B.* **5**, 1981, 40-51.

'Index to monumental inscriptions, Charlton Kings', *G.N.Q.* **1**, 1881, 121-3.

Cheltenham

ABHBA. 'Christ Church, Cheltenham: monumental inscriptions', *G.N.Q.* **4**, 1890, 604-12.

ABHBA. 'St. James Church, Cheltenham: monumental inscriptions', *G.N.Q.* **4**, 1890, 619-22.

ABHBA. 'St. Peter's Church, Cheltenham: monumental inscriptions', *G.N.Q.* **4**, 1890, 63-4.

BLACKER, BEAVER H. 'Monumental inscriptions in St. Peter's Church, Cheltenham, Gloucestershire', *Genealogist* **3**, 1879, 215-6. This is indexed in: 'Index to monumental inscriptions, St. Peter's, Cheltenham', *G.N.Q.* **1**, 1881, 42-3.

BLACKER, BEAVER H. *Monumental inscriptions in the parish church of Cheltenham, Gloucestershire*. Privately printed, 1877.

CHELTONIENSIS. 'Inscriptions in St. Mary's Cemetery, Cheltenham', *G.N.Q.* **3**, 1887, 425-32, 521-8, 608-15, and 651-63. 252 inscriptions.

CHELTONIENSIS. 'Inscriptions in the New Cemetery, near Cheltenham', *G.N.Q.* **4**, 1890, 305-16, and 365-73. 181 19th c. inscriptions relating to the parish of Cheltenham (although the cemetery is actually in Prestbury).

RAWES, J.A. *Memorial inscriptions of Cheltenham*. Lackhampton: the author, 1983 **1**: St. Mary's Church and churchyard. No more issued to date.

'Index to monumental inscriptions, Christ Church, Cheltenham', *G.N.Q.* **1**, 1888, 81-3.

'Index to monumental inscriptions, St. James's Church, Cheltenham', *G.N.Q.* **1**, 1881, 72-3.

'Index to monumental inscriptions, Trinity Church, Cheltenham', *G.N.Q.* **1**, 1881, 88-92, 96-7 and 101-3.

'Inscriptions in Cheltenham parish churchyard', *G.N.Q.* **2**, 1884, 607-11.

'Inscriptions in St Mary's cemetery, Cheltenham', *G.N.Q.* **3**, 1887, 425-32, 521-8, 608-15, and 651-63.

Chipping Campden

KNAPP, O.G. 'Campden brasses', *Evesham notes & queries* **3**, 1914, 225-30.

Chipping Campden Deanery

ROPER, IDA M. 'Monumental effigies: Rural Deanery of Chipping Campden', *B.G.A.S.Tr.* **32**, 1909, 219-59.

Chipping Sodbury

ABHBA. 'Chipping Sodbury church: monumental inscriptions', *G.N.Q.* **4**, 1890, 187-8.

Monumental Inscriptions: By Place continued

Cirencester
HADOW, W.E. 'On the monumental brasses at Cirencester', *B.G.A.S.Tr.* **2**, 1877/8, 151-62.
'[Inscriptions at St Johns, Cirencester]', *Gentleman's Magazine* **76**(1), 1806, 212-3.
See also Beckington.

Clifton
CAMPBELL, MARY V., ed. *Memorials of the church and churchyard of St. Andrews, Clifton.* 2 vols. Bristol: the editor, 1987.

Coates
See North Cerney.

Coombe Hill
COOPER, KEITH. 'Coombe Hill Methodist Church: index of names on memorials', *J.G.F.H.S.* **39**, 1988, 33.

Cranham
D., C.T. 'Cranham Church: monumental inscriptions', *G.N.Q.* **4**, 1890, 579-80.

Cromhall
ABHBA. 'Cromhall church: monumental inscriptions', *G.N.Q.* **4**, 1890, 644-7. See also **5**, 1894, 51.
VIATOR. 'Index to monumental inscriptions: Cromhall', *G.N.Q.* **3**, 1887, 211-13.

Cubberley
ABHBA. 'Cubberley church and church yard: monumental inscriptions', *G.N.Q.* **4**, 1890, 134-5.
BLACKER, BEAVER H. 'Monumental inscriptions at Cubberley, near Cheltenham, Gloucestershire', *Genealogist* **3**, 1879, 144.

Daglingworth, Driffield
See North Cerney.

Dursley Deanery
ROPER, IDA M. 'Monumental effigies: Dursley Rural Deanery', *B.G.A.S.Tr.* **29**, 1906, 147-63.

Edge
See Brimscombe.

Fairford
BIGLAND, R. *An account of the parish of Fairford, in the county of Gloucester: with a particular description of the stained glass in the windows of the church, engravings of ancient monuments.* J. Nichols, 1791. Includes monumental inscriptions, list of incumbents *etc.*
PARRY, H. 'Brasses in the church of St Mary, Fairford, Gloucestershire', *Somerset Archaeological & Natural History Society. Proceedings of the Bath & District Branch,* 1919-23, 166-7. Tame family.

Filton
ABHBA. 'Filton church: monumental inscriptions', *G.N.Q.* **4**, 1890, 461-2.
VIATOR. 'Index to monumental inscriptions, Filton', *G.N.Q.* **2**, 1884, 124.

Fishponds
ABHBA. 'Fishponds church: monumental inscriptions', *G.N.Q.* **4**, 1890, 462-3.
VIATOR. 'Index to monumental inscriptions: Fishponds', *G.N.Q.* **2**, 1884, 446-7.

Forest (North) Deanery
ROPER, IDA M. 'Monumental effigies: rural deanery of Forest (North)', *B.G.A.S.Tr.* **31**, 1908, 52-77.

Gloucester
BAZELEY, CANON, & MARGARET LEY. 'Effigies in Gloucester Cathedral', *B.G.A.S.Tr.* **27**, 1904, 289-326.

Gloucester Deanery
ROPER, IDA M. 'Monumental effigies: rural deanery of Gloucester', *B.G.A.S.Tr.* **31**, 1908, 207-43.

Great Witcombe
BLACKER, BEAVER H. 'Monumental inscriptions in the parish church, Great Witcombe, Gloucestershire', *Genealogist* **3**, 1879, 68-9.

Harescombe
'Monumental inscriptions, Harescombe', *G.N.Q.* **1**, 1881, 453-4.

Hatherop
See North Cerney.

Hawkesbury Deanery
ROPER, IDA M. 'Monumental effigies: rural Deanery of Hawkesbury', *B.G.A.S.Tr.* **30**, 1907, 123-41.

Hill
JENNER-FUST, H. 'Hill church: monumental inscriptions with notes', *G.N.Q.* **3**, 1887, 582-7.

King's Stanley
'Monumental inscriptions, King's Stanley', *G.N.Q.* **1**, 1881, 171-3.
ADHBA. 'Stanley Kings church: monumental inscriptions', *G.N.Q.* **4**, 1890, 473-7.

Kingswood
ABHBA. 'Trinity Church, Kingswood: monumental inscriptions', *G.N.Q.* **4**, 1890, 273.

Leckhampton
PINK, W.D. 'Inscriptions in Leckhampton church', *G.N.Q.* **5**, 1894, 449-51.
'Index to monumental inscriptions, Leckhampton', *G.N.Q.* **1**, 1881, 60-62, and 67-8.

Monumental Inscriptions: By Place continued

Leigh
'The Leigh, Gloucestershire: monumental inscriptions', *J.G.F.H.S.* **6**, 1980, 9. Surnames only.

Leonard Stanley
ABHBA. 'Stanley St. Leonards church: monumental inscriptions', *G.N.Q.* **4**, 1890, 477-82.
'Index to monumental inscriptions, Stanley St. Leonards', *G.N.Q.* **1**, 1881, 409-10.

Longney
ABHBA. 'Longney Church: monumental inscriptions', *G.N.Q.* **4**, 1890, 80-82.
BLACKER, BEAVER H. 'Monumental inscriptions in the parish church, Longney, Gloucestershire.' *Genealogist* **3**, 1879, 214-5.
'Index to monumental inscriptions, Longney', *G.N.Q.* **1**, 1881, 42.

Maisemore
DIGHTON, CONWAY. 'Maisemore church: monumental inscriptions', *G.N.Q.* **4**, 1890, 274-84.

Miserden
'Index to monumental inscriptions, Miserden', *G.N.Q.* **1**, 1881, 300-301.

Nailsworth
See Brimscombe.

North Cerney
DRUITT, H. 'Gloucestershire notes', *Monumental Brass Society transactions* **5**, 1906, 159-60. Inscriptions at North Cerney, Coates, Daglingworth, Driffield, Hatherop and Sapperton.

Northleach
'[Inscriptions on tombs in Northleach church]', *Gentleman's magazine*, **76**(1), 1806. 213-4.

Northleach Deanery
ROPER, IDA M. 'Monumental effigies: rural deanery of Northleach', *B.G.A.S.Tr.* **33**, 1910, 96-125.

Oakridge
ABHBA. 'Oakridge church: monumental inscriptions', *G.N.Q.* **4**, 1890, 460-1.
See also Brimscombe.

Oldbury on the Hill
LEWIN, R.A. 'Monumental inscriptions in Avon, Gloucestershire and Somerset', *J.B.A.* **3**, 1976, 9-14. Includes summary of inscriptions from Oldbury on the Hill, Glos.

Painswick
DAVIS, CECIL T. 'Monumental inscriptions at Painswick, Co. Gloucester', *M.G.H.*, 4th series **1**, 1904-5, 276-7.
G., J. 'Index to monumental inscriptions, Painswick', *G.N.Q.* **1**, 1881, 180-1, and 188-91.
MANSFIELD, GWEN. 'Painswick', *J.G.F.H.S.* **11**, 1981, 5-6. Includes list of monumental inscriptions.
MANSFIELD, GWEN. 'Painswick, 1981', *J.G.F.H.S.* **9**, 1981, 16. List of 9 monumental inscriptions remaining at Friends' Meeting House.

Pitchcombe
ABHBA. 'Pitchcombe church: monumental inscriptions', *G.N.Q.* **4**, 1890, 420-5.
'Index to monumental inscriptions, Pitchcombe', *G.N.Q.* **1**, 1881, 56-7.

Postlip
RAWES, JULIAN. 'St. James Chapel, Postlip', *J.G.F.H.S.* **32**, 1987, 21. Roman Catholic monumental inscriptions.

Prestbury
BLACKER, BEAVER H. 'Monumental inscriptions in the parish church, Prestbury', *Genealogist* **2**, 1878, 259-62.
See also Cheltenham.

Randwick
ABHBA. 'Randwick parish church: monumental inscriptions', *G.N.Q.* **4**, 1890, 543-7.
MANSFIELD, GWEN. 'Monumental inscriptions in the graveyard of Randwick Methodist Chapel', *J.G.F.H.S.* **16**, 1983, 11. Surnames only.
'Index to monumental inscriptions *etc.*, Randwick', *G.N.Q.* **1**, 1881, 144-6.

Redland
ABHBA. 'Redland Green chapel, Bristol: monumental inscriptions', *G.N.Q.* **4**, 1890, 411-16. Also includes inscriptions from Backwell, Somerset.
VIATOR. 'Index to monumental inscriptions: Redland Green chapel, Bristol', *G.N.Q.* **2**, 1884, 489-91, and **4**, 1890, 411-15. In Westbury on Trym parish; includes transcripts.
WILKINS, H.J. *Redland Chapel and Redland*. Bristol: J.W. Arrowsmith, 1924. Includes monumental inscriptions and list of ministers.

Rockhampton
'Notes on Rockhampton parish', *G.N.Q.* **3**, 1887, 536-43. Includes monumental inscriptions, list of rectors, 1386-1886, and extracts from the parish register *etc.*

Monumental Inscriptions: By Place continued

Rockhampton *continued*
ABHBA. 'Further notes on Rockhampton parish', *G.N.Q.* **4**, 1890, 586-96. Includes further monumental inscriptions, extracts from churchwardens accounts *etc.*

Rodborough
ABHBA. 'Rodborough church: monumental inscriptions', *G.N.Q.* **4**, 1890, 515-9.
'Index to monumental inscriptions, Rodborough', *G.N.Q.* **1**, 1881, 50-2.

Sapperton
ABHBA. 'Sapperton monumental inscriptions', *G.N.Q.* **4**, 1890, 346-9.
RAWES, JULIAN. 'Sapperton cemetery, Sapperton, Gloucestershire', *J.G.F.H.S.* **35**, 1987, 27.
'Index to monumental inscriptions, Sapperton', *G.N.Q.* **1**, 1881, 316-7.
See also North Cerney.

Sheepscombe
See Brimscombe.

Shirehampton
ADHBA. 'Shirehampton Church: monumental inscriptions', *G.N.Q.* **4**, 1890, 181-2.
'Index to monumental inscriptions, Shirehampton', *G.N.Q.* **2**, 1884, 392-3.

Slade
See Brimscombe.

Stanley Kings
See King's Stanley.

Stanley St. Leonard's
See Leonard Stanley.

Stonehouse
ABHBA. 'Stonehouse church: monumental inscriptions', *G.N.Q.* **4**, 1890, 449-56.
S., C.L. 'St. Cyril's Church, Stonehouse', *G.N.Q.* **7**, 1900, 163-7, and 179-84. Includes monumental inscriptions *etc*.
'Index to monumental inscriptions, Stonehouse', *G.N.Q.* **1**, 1881, 128-9.

Stonehouse Deanery
SMITH, WINIFRED F. 'Monumental effigies: deanery of Stonehouse', *B.G.A.S.Tr.* **28**, 1905, 94-106. For erratum, see **29**, 1906, end paper.

Stow Deanery
WITTS, E.J.B. 'Monumental effigies, Rural Deanery of Stow', *B.G.A.S.Tr.* **28**, 1905, 107-10.

Stroud
G., J. 'Rodborough tabernacle; monumental inscriptions *etc*.', *G.N.Q.* **2**, 1884, 60-62. At Stroud.
'Monumental inscriptions at Stroud (St. Lawrence)', *J.G.F.H.S.* **13**, 1982, 10-11. Surnames only.

Swindon
ABHBA. 'Swindon Church: monumental inscriptions', *G.N.Q.* **4**, 1890, 155-8, and 167-9.
BLACKER, BEAVER H. 'Monumental inscriptions in the parish church of Swindon, Gloucestershire', *Genealogist* **1**, 1877, 332-3 and 366-8. This is indexed in: 'Index to monumental inscriptions, Swindon', *G.N.Q.* **1**, 1881, 46-7.
WYLLMER. 'Swindon and its church', *G.N.Q.* **7**, 1900, 1-6 and 69-80. Includes monumental inscriptions, list of rectors *etc*.

Tewkesbury
LYSONS, SAMUEL. 'Observations on some of the tombs in the abbey church at Tewkesbury', *Archaeologia* **14**, 1803, 143-53.
RAWES, JULIAN. 'Memorial inscriptions: Tewkesbury Baptist Chapel, Barton Street, Tewkesbury', *J.G.F.H.S.* **38**, 1988, 10.
RAWES, J.A. 'Monumental inscriptions at Holy Trinity, Tewkesbury', *J.G.F.H.S.* **12**, 1982, 19. Surnames only.
SYMONDS, W.S. 'Historical notes on some of the tombs in Tewkesbury Abbey', *B.G.A.S.Tr.* **2**, 1877/8, 194-209.

Turkdean
TUDOR, J.L. 'Monumental inscriptions in Turkdean parish church', *G.N.Q.* **2**, 1884, 226-9.

Westbury on Trym
See Redland.

Winchcombe Deanery
ROPER, IDA M. 'Monumental effigies: rural deanery of Winchcombe', *B.G.A.S.Tr.* **29**, 1906, 230-64.

Woodchester
ABHBA. 'Woodchester church: monumental inscriptions *etc*.', *G.N.Q.* **4**, 1890, 352-8.
'Index to monumental inscriptions, Woodchester', *G.N.Q.* **1**, 1881, 152-4.

Wotton under Edge
CORDWELL, J.E. 'Wotton under Edge: surnames on churchyard inscriptions', *J.G.F.H.S.* **5**, 1980, 21-4. List of surnames from St Mary the Virgin, the Baptist Church, and the Tabernacle.

Yate
ABHBA. 'Yate Church: monumental inscriptions', *G.N.Q.* **4**, 1890, 196-9.

Monumental Inscriptions continued

C. BY FAMILY

Adams
See Lyde and Wills.

Africanus
See Wills.

Berkeley
BAGNALL-OAKLEY, MARY ELLEN. 'On the monumental effigies of the family of Berkeley', *B.G.A.S.Tr.* **15**, 1890-1, 89-102.
PHILLIMORE, W.P.W. 'Cranford and the Berkeleys', *G.N.Q.* **4**, 1890, 665-67. Monumental inscriptions at Cranford, Middlesex, relating to the Berkeleys of Gloucestershire.

Bovey
'Mrs Catherine Bovey, of Flaveley Manor: her monumental inscriptions', *G.N.Q.* **1**, 1881, 340-42. 1727.

Bray
'Bray monument in Great Barrington Church', *G.N.Q.* **1**, 1881, 358-9. 17-18th c.

Clopton
MACLEAN, SIR JOHN. 'Notes on a monumental effigy and a "brass" in the church of Quinton, Gloucestershire', *B.G.A.S.Tr.* **3**, 1888-9, 162-72. Clopton family.

Codrington
C., R.H. 'The tomb of John Codrington', *G.N.Q.* **7**, 1900, 143-6, 147-5. Includes brief genealogical notes.

Cornock
GODDARD, R.W.K. 'Cornock, monuments at Berkeley and Nibley', *G.N.Q.* **6**, 1896, 31-2 and 97-8; **7**, 1900, 96-8.

Foster
See Lyde.

Fowler
'Edward Fowler, D.D., Bishop of Gloucester: his monumental inscription', *G.N.Q.* **3**, 1887, 225-6.

Freeman
P[OWELL], J.J. 'Freeman inscriptions, Hempsted and Bushley', *G.N.Q.* **3**, 1887, 150-52.

Graile
'Thomas Graile, rector of Lassington', *G.N.Q.* **2**, 1884, 380-1. Graile family inscriptions.

Gregory
See Wood.

Holbrow
'The Holbrow family', *G.N.Q.* **1**, 1881, 233-4. Monumental inscriptions.

Jenkinson
FOLJAMBE, CECIL G.S. 'The Jenkinson monuments in Hawkesbury Church', *G.N.Q.* **5**, 1894, 252-60.

Jones
GRAY, I.E. 'The iconography of archives, IV: the monument of John Jones at Gloucester', *Journal of the Society of Archivists* **3**, 1965-9, 488-9. 1630.

Kelke
EARWAKER, JOHN P. 'Clement Kelke: his monumental inscription', *G.N.Q.* **2**, 1884, 18. 1593.

Lond
BOUCHER, C.E. 'The Lond or Loud brass in St Peter's Church, Bristol', *B.G.A.S.Tr.* **30**, 1907, 265-9.

Lyde
'Lyde, Foster and Adams inscriptions, Stanton Drew', *G.N.Q.* **3**, 1887, 161-3.

Merrett
R., F.L.M. 'The Merrett family', *G.N.Q.* **5**, 1894, 106. Monumental inscriptions, 17th c.

Mitchell
See Muir.

Muir
COOPER, KEITH. 'The Postlip burial enclosure', *J.G.F.H.S.* **37**, 1988, 5. Muir and Mitchell family inscriptions, 20th c.

Newland
B[LACKER], B.H. 'Inscriptions on flat stone in parish church of Painswick, Gloucestershire', *Genealogist* **6**, 1882, 315. Newland family.

Partridge
D., C.T. 'The Partridge family: monumental inscriptions', *G.N.Q.* **2**, 1884, 180-1.

Paul
'The Paul family', *G.N.Q.* **1**, 1881, 352-6. See also 439. Monumental inscriptions.

Pettat
'The Pettat family', *G.N.Q.* **1**, 1881, 208-10. Monumental inscriptions.

Porter
'The Porter family of Bristol: monumental inscriptions', *G.N.Q.* **3**, 1887, 30-34. See also 59-61.

Pouldon
'Pouldon and Whitmore families', *G.N.Q.* **2**, 1884, 634-5. Monumental inscriptions.

Monumental Inscriptions: By Family continued

Robins
T., H.Y.J. 'The Robins family', *G.N.Q.* **5**, 1894, 13. Monumental inscriptions to Anne Robins, 1732.

Saintloe
See Wood.

Semys
DAVIS, CECIL T. 'Brass at St. John Baptist, Gloucester', *G.N.Q.* **5**, 1894, 539-45. To John Semys, 16th c.

Sly
PAINTER, A.C. 'An inscription at Chedworth', *B.G.A.S.Tr.* **55**, 1933, 143-9. Richard Sly, 1461.

Snigge
BRISTOLIENSIS. 'Sir George Snigge's monument in St Stephens, Bristol', *G.N.Q.* **4**, 1890, 299-300. 1617.

Stratford
ROPER, IDA M. 'Effigies of the Stratford family at Farmcote, Gloucestershire', *B.G.A.S.Tr.* **49**, 1927, 277-80.

Whitmore
See Pouldon.

Wills
VIATOR. 'Three inscriptions in Henbury churchyard', *G.N.Q.* **2**, 1894, 123. Wills, Africanus, and Adams memorials.

Wilson
ROPER, IDA M. & HUDLESTON, C. ROY. 'A sixteenth century monument in Westbury on Trym church', *B.G.A.S.Tr.* **53**, 1931, 207-14. Miles Wilson, 1567.

Winston
MAYO, CHARLES H. 'The Winston monument in Long Barton church, Dorset', *G.N.Q.* **2**, 1884, 157-8. Of Standish, Gloucestershire.

Wood
D., G. 'Three monumental inscriptions from Oxford', *G.N.Q.* **4**, 1890, 399-400. Richard Wood, 1598; John Gregory, 1695. Mary Saintloe, 1699.

Woodward
'The Woodward family: monumental inscriptions', *G.N.Q.* **2**, 1884, 79-80.

Young
WERE, F. 'Monument to, and heraldry of Sir John and Dame Yonge (Young) in Bristol Cathedral', *B.G.A.S.Tr.* **35**(1), 1912, 935.

11. OFFICIAL LISTS OF NAMES

Governments are keen on listing their subjects, a trait for which genealogists have cause to be thankful, since the lists which result enable us to locate precisely our ancestors in time and place. Official lists have been compiled for a multitude of reasons: taxation, defence, voting, land ownership *etc*. A useful general discussion of Gloucestershire fiscal records is provided by:

ELRINGTON, CHRISTOPHER R. 'Assessment of Gloucestershire: fiscal records in local history', *B.G.A.S.Tr.* **103**, 1985, 5-15.

Domesday book provides the earliest general listing of manorial lords, and has recently been re-published:

MOORE, JOHN S., ed. *Domesday book, 15: Gloucestershire*. Phillimore: Chichester, 1982. A useful genealogical analysis of Domesday book, including many pedigrees, is:

ELLIS, ALFRED S. 'On the landholders of Gloucestershire named in Domesday Book', *B.G.A.S.Tr.* **4**, 1879-80, 86-198.

A number of works provide useful information from medieval fiscal records. They are listed here chronologically:

BARKLY, SIR HENRY. 'Remarks on the liber niger, or black book, of the Exchequer', *B.G.A.S.Tr.* **14**, 1889-90, 285-320. Notes on Knights fees, 1166.

BARKLY, SIR HENRY. 'Kirkby's quest', *B.G.A.S.Tr.* **11**, 1886-7, 130-54. List of knights fees held, late 13th c.

BARKLY, SIR HENRY. 'Testa de Nevill: return for the county of Gloucester', *B.G.A.S.Tr.* **12**, 1887-8, 235-90; **13**, 1888-9, 23-34 and 297-358; **14**, 1889-90, 14-47. 1302. Includes many biographical notes.

BARKLY, SIR HENRY. 'Testa de Nevill, with an attempt to determine the dates of the returns pertaining to the county of Gloucester contained therein', *Genealogist* N.S. **5**, 1889, 35-40, and 75-80.

HALL, J. MELLAND. 'A list of Gloucestershire knights, 1323-4', *G.N.Q.* **2**, 1884, 367. From writs of military summons.

MACLEAN, SIR JOHN. 'The aid levied in Gloucestershire in 20th Edw. III (1349)', *B.G.A.S.Tr.* **10**, 1885-6, 278-92.

MACLEAN, SIR JOHN. 'Knights fees in Gloucestershire, 3rd Henry IV', *B.G.A.S.Tr.* **11**, 1886-7, 312-30. 1401-2.

Official Lists of Names continued

Taxation Lists
From the medieval period until the seventeenth century, the subsidy provided one of the main sources of government income. This role was taken over by the hearth tax after the Restoration. Unfortunately, only one tax roll covering the whole county has been published – and that is an edition which is now very rare: *Gloucestershire subsidy roll, 1 Edward III, A.D. 1327*. [Middle Hill: Sir Thomas Phillipps, 1856?]
A general list of those gentry responsible for collecting an assessment in 1657 is provided by:
EARWAKER, J.P. 'Names of Gloucestershire gentry in 1657', *G.N.Q.* **2**, 1884, 91-2. Lists of commissions for collecting the assessment of 1657.

Many subsidy rolls and other tax lists relating to particular places have been published. See:

Bisley
'Subsidy roll for Bisley, 1600', *G.N.Q.* **3**, 1887, 5-6.

Bisley Hundred
'Bisley and Longtree hundreds: duties upon houses, windows, and lights 1774', *G.N.Q.* **2**, 1884, 92-3. Presumably lists collectors.

Bristol
FULLER, E.A. 'The tallage of Edward II (Dec 16, 1312) and the Bristol rebellion', *B.G.A.S.Tr.* **19**, 1894-5, 171-278. Bristol tax list; also includes Bristol subsidy, 1327.
GIBSON, J.S.W. 'Bristol tax assessments in the later Stuart period (1660-1715)', *J.B.A.* **37**, 1984, 21-5. General discussion of tax lists relating to the subsidy, hearth tax and land tax *etc.*, held at Bristol Record Office.
GIBSON, J.S.W. 'The hearth tax in Bristol', *J.B.A.* **36**, 1984, 9-13. Describes the 'chimney book, 1665-72', held at Bristol Record Office. No names, but essential guide to a valuable source. Also lists hearth tax rolls at P.R.O. for Bristol.
RALPH, ELIZABETH. 'A Bristol poll tax 1666', *B.G.A.S.Tr.* **61**, 1939, 178-87.
RALPH, ELIZABETH, & WILLIAMS, MARY E., eds. *The inhabitants of Bristol in 1696*. Bristol Record Society publications **25**. Bristol: the Society, 1968. Return under the Marriage Duty Act, 1694.

Brookthorpe
HALL, J. MELLAND. 'Brockthorp taxpayers, 1327-1584', *G.N.Q.* **3**, 1887, 92-3. Subsidy rolls, 1327, 1557/8, and 1584.

Cam
PHILLIMORE, W.P.W. 'The parish of Cam, 1571', *G.N.Q.* **2**, 1881, 113. Lay subsidy.

Charlton Kings
GREET, M.J. 'Charlton Kings and the hundred of Cheltenham in 1327: a note on the lay subsidy roll for 1 Edward III', *C.K.L.H.S.B.* **7**, 1982, 35-7. Gives names.

Cranham
H., J.M. 'Poll tax (parish of Cranham), temp., Rich. II', *G.N.Q.* **3**, 1887, 277-8.

Elmore
GUISE, WILLIAM V. 'Subsidy roll for Elmore parish, 1327', *G.N.Q.* **2**, 1884, 155-6.

Haresfield
HALL, J. MELLAND. 'Subsidy roll for Haresfield, 1327', *G.N.Q.* **2**, 1884, 270-1.

Longtree Hundred
See Bisley Hundred.

Olveston
HAINES, ROBERT J. 'The hearth tax returns for Olveston, Gloucestershire, 1671', *J.B.A.* **26**, 1981, 28-9.

Uley
PHILLIMORE, W.P.W. 'The parish of Uley, 1571', *G.N.Q.* **2**, 1884, 39. Lay subsidy roll, listing 10 tax payers.

Defence of the Realm
Another reason for compiling lists was the defence of the realm. Contributors for this purpose are listed in:
'Gloucestershire and the Spanish Armada', *G.N.Q.* **1**, 1881, 440-42.
The defence of the realm necessitated the involvement of everyone fit to bear arms, *i.e.*, every adult male. In 1608, everyone appearing at musters was listed in a volume which is now perhaps the most important published listing of Gloucestershire's inhabitants genealogically speaking:
SMITH, JOHN. *Men and armor for Gloucestershire in 1608*. Gloucester: Alan Sutton, 1980. Originally published as *The names and surnames of all the able and sufficient men in body fit for His Majesty's service in the wars within the county of Gloucester*. Sotheran, 1902.

Official Lists of Names:
Defence of the Realm *continued*

The classic analysis of this list deserves mention, although it has little direct bearing on genealogy:

TAWNEY, A.J. & R.H. 'An occupational census of the seventeenth century', *Economic History review* **5**, 1934, 25-64.

See also:

MACLEAN, JOHN. 'Smyth's Mss: book of array, 1608', *G.N.Q.* **2**, 1884, 627-34. Muster list for the Forest of Dean.

Notes on musters in the early seventeenth century are also included amongst the lieutenancy papers of the Earl of Hertford, Lord Lieutenant of Bristol, as well as of Wiltshire and Somerset:

MURPHY, W.P.D., ed. *The Earl of Hertford's lieutenancy papers, 1603-1612*. Wiltshire Record Society **23**. Devizes: the Society, 1969.

Poll Books and Electoral Registers

When parliamentary elections were contested lists of those claiming the right to vote were sometimes published, showing how they exercised that right. Before the reform of 1832 contested elections for the County (for which 40s. freeholders had the franchise) were rare, as the opposing parties usually came to a prior agreement in order to avoid excessive cost. Copies of printed poll books for 1714/5, 1776 and 1811 survive in a few libraries only. For Bristol they are more numerous, and there are occasional published polls for Cirencester, Gloucester and Tewkesbury (probably for a very restricted franchise). After 1832 (until the introduction of the secret vote in 1872) they are more numerous, and there are also annual electoral registers, of which one or more sets appear to survive virtually unbroken. Details of these and the location of surviving copies are given in works cited in *English genealogy: an introductory bibliography*, chapter 12, D. See also:

AUSTIN, ROLAND. 'Gloucestershire poll-books', *Notes & queries*, 10th series **10**, 1908, 124. This is now very out of date, and reference should also be made to Austin's *Catalogue*, (above, p.9), as well as to *English genealogy*.

The only modern published polling lists are:

HUDLESTON, C. ROY. 'Gloucestershire voters in 1710', *B.G.A.S.Tr.* **58**, 1936, 195-205. Covers Langley and Swineshead hundreds only; and that published with the parish register of St. Augustine the Less, Bristol (above, page 36).

Census Returns

By far the most useful lists are those deriving from the official censuses. These began in 1801, but the earliest surviving returns of genealogical value are those for 1841. Two earlier, unofficial censuses were, however, compiled, and have been published:

DOWNEND LOCAL HISTORY SOCIETY. 'The inhabitants of Mangotsfield parish, May 2, 1798', *J.B.A.* **7**, 1977, 23.

HAINES, ROBERT J. 'The inhabitants of Olveston, Gloucestershire, in 1742', *J.B.A.* **15**, 1979, 18-22. List of 125 households.

Works on the official census in Gloucestershire are few. The most useful is the index to the 1851 census for Bristol:

1851 census for Bristol and Avon. Bristol: Bristol & Avon Family History Society, 1987-88. **1**. Bedminster, St. Paul. **2**. St. Stephen, St. Thomas and St. John the Baptist. **3**. St. Nicholas, Christ Church, and Castle Precincts. **4**. Temple. **5**. St. Mary Redcliffe. **6**. St. Augustine the Less.

See also:

WATTS, JOHN. 'Enumeration district maps', *J.B.A.* **41**, 1985, 26-31. Discussion of Bristol districts.

BAKER, JANE. 'Bristol census returns 1851, 1861, 1871', *J.B.A.* **42**, 1985, 28-30. Description of registration districts.

BATES, CHRISTOPHER. 'Bristol girls at t'mill', *J.B.A.* **11**, 1978, 15-16. Extracts from 1851 census of Ellen Holme, Sowerby and Halifax, Yorkshire.

'St. Peter's Hospital, Bristol: 1851 census', *J.B.A.* **61**, 1990, 17-20. List of 188 staff and patients.

BAKER, JANE. 'Bristol census 1881: an outline', *J.B.A.* **48**, 1987, 37-8. Lists census returns on microfilm.

12. DIRECTORIES AND MAPS

Directories are an invaluable source of information for locating people in the past. For the nineteenth century, they are the equivalent of the modern phone book. Many directories for Gloucestershire were published. The list which follows is selective, largely based on volumes I have actually seen in Bristol or Gloucester, although also drawing on information from the works listed in Chapter 13 of *English genealogy: an introductory bibliography*. Austin's *Catalogue* (above, p.9) also provides many references. The list which follows is in chronological order.

TUNNICLIFF, WILLIAM. *A topographical survey of the counties of Somerset, Gloucester, Worcester, Stafford, Chester and Lancaster*. R. Cruttwell, 1789.

GELL, R., & BRADSHAW, T. *The Gloucestershire directory, containing the names and residences of professional gentlemen, merchants, manufacturers and tradesmen in Gloucester, Cheltenham, Cirencester, Tewkesbury, Stroud, Wotton under Edge, Dursley, Tetbury, Painswick, etc...* Gloucester: J. Roberts, 1820.

Hunt & Co's City of Gloucester and Cheltenham directory and court guide ... [also] ... surrounding villages ... E. Hunt & Co., 1847.

Hunt & Co's directory and topography for the cities of Gloucester and Bristol and the towns of Berkeley, Cirencester ... [etc.] E. Hunt & Co., 1849.

Post Office directory of Gloucestershire with Bath and Bristol. Kelly & Co., 1856-1939. 18 issues. Title varies; sometimes referred to as *Kelly's directory of the county of Gloucester*.

Harrison, Harrod & Co's *Bristol Post Office directory and gazetteer, with the counties of Gloucestershire and Somerset ...* Thomas Danks for Harrison, Harrod & Co., 1859.

Morris & Co's commercial directory and gazetteer of Gloucestershire with Bristol and Monmouth. Nottingham: Morris & Co., 1865-76. 3 issues.

Slaters (late Pigot & Co.) royal national and commercial directory and topography of the counties of Gloucestershire, Monmouthshire, and North and South Wales, and a classified directory of the town of Liverpool ... Isaac Slater, 1858-9.

Harmer's Cotswold almanack and trade directory, for 1868, comprising the calendar, a guide and directory for Cirencester, Fairford, Cricklade, Lechlade, Tetbury, Malmesbury and Northleach

W.E. Owen & Co's general topographical and historical directory for Gloucestershire, Wiltshire, Somersetshire, Monmouthshire, Radnorshire, with the cities of Bristol and Bath. Leicester: W.E. Owen & Co., 1879.

Deacon's court guide, gazetteer and royal blue book: a fashionable register ... of the county of Gloucester. C.W. Deacon & Co., 1880. Continued by: *The Gloucester court guide and county blue book*. C.W. Deacon & Co., 1899.

Gloucestershire directory and buyers' guide. Walsall: E.F. Cope & Co., 1910-36. 4 issues. Continued by *Gloucestershire and Bristol directory*. Walsall: Aubrey & Co., 1937-40. 3 issues.

Bristol

Sketchley's Bristol directory, 1775. Bath: Kingsmead Reprints, 1971. Originally published Bristol: James Sketchley, 1775.

'Montague Street, Kingsdown', *J.B.A.* **47**, 1987, 30-31. List of residents from Sketchley's Bristol directory, 1775.

The Bristol directory ... containing an alphabetical list of the names and places of abode of the principal inhabitants, merchants, tradesmen, manufacturers, etc. of the city of Bristol and its environs, including Bedminster, Clifton, and the Hot Wells

BAILEY, WILLIAM. *The Bristol and Bath directory ...* Bristol: W. Routh, 1787.

REED, JOHN. *The new Bristol directory for ... 1792 ...* Bristol: Wm. Browne *et al.*, 1792.

Matthews' new Bristol directory for the year 17–, containing an alphabetical list of the Corporation, clergy, merchants, bankers, professors of the law and physics, manufacturers, principal traders, etc., etc., of the City of Bristol ... Bristol: William Matthews, 1793-1857. Annual; title varies. 1st edition also published as MATTHEWS, WILLIAM. *The new history, survey, and description of the city and suburbs of Bristol ...* Bristol: William Matthews, 1794. Continued by: *Matthews' annual directory for the city and county of Bristol, including Clifton, Bedminster and surrounding villages*. Matthew Matthews, 1858-69, *Matthews' Bristol directory with adjacent villages, remodelled by J.Wright*. Bristol: J. Wright & Co., 1870-79, and *J. Wright & Co's Bristol and Clifton directory with nearly 100 adjacent villages*. Bristol: J. Wright, 1880-1923. Annual to 1917; 3 issues thereafter. Published by Kelly's from 1904, in place of their *Kelly's directory of the City of Bristol and suburbs*. Kelly & Co., 1889-1950. 25 issues.

Directories and Maps: Bristol continued

The Bristol index, or Evans' directory ... Bristol: John Evans & Co., 1816-18. 3 issues; 1818 ed. published by Browne & Manchee.

Hunt & Co's ... Bristol, Clifton and Hotwells directory ... *1848*. B.W. Gardiner for E. Hunt & Co., 1848.

Hunt & Co's directory and topography for the city of Bristol, Bedminster, Clifton, Hotwells ... also the towns of Axbridge, Burnham, Clevedon and Weston Super Mare. E. Hunt & Co., 1850.

Post Office directory of Somerset and Bristol. Kelly & Co., 1861-83. 3 eds.

The Clifton and Redland directory for 1891 ... Bristol: William F. Mack, 1891.

The New Bristol directory. Bristol: Sharp & Co., 1903-5. Continued by: *Sharp's Bristol directory, incorporating the new Bristol directory*. Bristol: Sharp & Co., 1906.

Cheltenham

Cheltenham directory, 18–, comprehending a list of the principal inhabitants, tradesmen and lodging houses ... Cheltenham: W. Buckle, 1800-1802. 2 issues.

The Cheltenham annuaire ... Cheltenham: H. Davies, 1837-99. Annual. Continued by *The Cheltenham and Gloucestershire directory*. Cheltenham: H. Davies, 1900-1912. Despite the title, this only relates to Cheltenham.

The original Cheltenham directory for 1839. Cheltenham: T.E. Weller, 1839. Also referred to as *Weller's original Cheltenham directory*.

Rowe's illustrated Cheltenham guide. Cheltenham: George Rowe, 1845.

Harper's commercial and fashionable guide for Cheltenham and the adjoining hamlets. Cheltenham: S.C. Harper, 1843-4. 2 issues. Continued by: *Harper's Cheltenham directory, 18–* . Cheltenham: A. Harper, 1853-7. 2 issues.

Edwards' new Cheltenham directory for 18–. Cheltenham: R. Edwards, 1848-62. 5 issues. Continued by: *The Royal Cheltenham directory, 18–*. Cheltenham: Richard Edwards, 1870-78 (7 issues, little varies), and by *The Cheltenham Post Office directory*. Cheltenham: Horace Edwards, 1880-92. 3 issues.

Kelly's directory of Cheltenham with Charlton Kings, Leckhampton and Prestbury. Kelly's Directories, 1926-1950. Almost annually.

Forest of Dean

G.J. Harris's Forest of Dean directory and almanack for 18–. Lydney: G.J. Harris, 1892-1914. 9 issues.

Gloucester

The Gloucester new guide ... Gloucester: R. Raikes, 1802.

A directory of the city of Gloucester for 1841. Gloucester: Lewis Bryant, 1841.

Hunt & Co's city of Gloucester, and Cheltenham directory and court guide ... E. Hunt & Co., 1847. Only Gloucester and Cheltenham.

Hunt & Co's commercial directory for the cities of Gloucester, Hereford and Worcester ... E. Hunt & Co., 1847.

Bretherton's almanack and Gloucester directory for 18– . Gloucester: D. Bretherton, 1862-82. Annual.

The city of Gloucester diary, directory and almanack for 18–. Gloucester: L.A. Smart, 1883-7. Annual. Continued by: *Smart's City of Gloucester and district directory of names, residences and general local information*. Gloucester: L.A. Smart, 1889-1936. 13 issues.

Stroud

The New directory of Stroud and district, 1908. Stroud: Harry Harmer, 1908-9. 2 issues.

Directories sometimes, usefully, include maps, which you will need to consult in order to locate particular places. Early maps reveal a great deal about the way in which the landscape has changed in modern times. A number have been recently reprinted:

A Gloucestershire and Bristol atlas: a selection of old maps and plans from the 16th to the 19th c., including the Isaac Taylor (1777) large scale map of the county in full. B.G.A.S., 1961.

LOBEL, M.D., ed. *The atlas of historic towns, vol. 2: Bristol, Cambridge, Coventry, Norwich*. Scolar Press, 1975.

The old series Ordnance Survey maps of England and Wales ... *vol. **IV**: Central England*. Lympne Castle: Harry Margary, 1986.

Individual sheet maps of the 1st edition O.S. maps have been reprinted by the publishers David & Charles.

Many early maps are listed in:

CHUBB, T. *A descriptive catalogue of the printed maps of Gloucestershire, 1577-1911, with biographical notes*. Bristol: Bristol & Gloucestershire Archaeological Society, 1912. Supplement to *B.G.A.S.Tr*. **35**, 1912. See also AUSTIN, ROBERT. 'Additions to Mr. Chubb's *Descriptive catalogue* ...', *B.G.A.S.Tr*. **39**, 1916, 233-64.

13. RELIGIOUS RECORDS

The role of the church in society was formerly much greater than it is today. Consequently, many of the sources essential to the genealogist are to be found in ecclesiastical rather than state archives – for example, parish registers, probate records, local government records *etc*. Works on ecclesiastical sources are to be found throughout this bibliography; this chapter concentrates on those topics which are primarily to do with the administration of the church. General background to medieval ecclesiastical history is provided by:

HAINES, P.M. *The administration of the Diocese of Worcester in the first half of the fourteenth century*. S.P.C.K., 1965.

The most important ecclesiastical sources for the medieval period are the bishops' registers. These record the general business of the diocese. The lists of ordinations and institutions they contain, together with the occasional will, are of particular value to genealogists. In this period, Gloucestershire was an archdeaconry within the diocese of Worcester. Published registers include:

BUND, J.W. WILLIS, ed. *Episcopal registers, Diocese of Worcester: register of Bishop Godfrey Giffard, September 23rd, 1268 to January 26th, 1302*. 2 vols. Oxford: James Parker & Co., for the Worcestershire Historical Society, 1898-1902.

BUND, J.W. WILLIS, ed. *The register of the Diocese of Worcester during the vacancy of the see, usually called 'registrum sede vacante'*. 5 vols. Oxford: James Parker & Co., for the Worcestershire Historical Society, 1893-7. 1301-1435.

BUND, J.W. WILLIS, ed. *Register of Bishop William Ginsborough, 1303 to 1307*. Oxford: James Parker & Co., 1907.

PEARCE, ERNEST HAROLD, ed. *The register of Thomas de Cobham, Bishop of Worcester, 1317-1327*. Mitchell Hughes & Clarke, for the Worcestershire Historical Society, 1930.

MARETT, WARWICK PAUL, ed. *A calendar of the register of Henry Wakefield, Bishop of Worcester, 1375-95*. Worcestershire Historical Society, N.S. **7**. Leeds: the Society, 1972.

SMITH, WALDO E.L., ed. *The register of Richard Clifford, Bishop of Worcester, 1401-1407: a calendar*. Subsidia mediaevalia **6**. Toronto: Pontifical Institute of Mediaeval Studies, 1976.

Many papers relating to ecclesiastical administration in the twelfth century are printed in:

MOREY, ADRIAN, & BROOKE, CHRISTOPHER NUGENT LAWRENCE, eds. *The letters and charters of Gilbert Foliot, abbot of Gloucester (1139-48), bishop of Hereford (1148-63) and London (1163-87)*. Cambridge: Cambridge University Press, 1967.

Lists of the medieval archdeacons of Gloucester are to be found in:

LE NEVE, JOHN. *Fasti ecclesiae Anglicanae, 1066-1300. Vol.2: Monastic cathedrals (northern and southern provinces)*, comp. Diana E. Greenway. Athlone Press, 1971.

LE NEVE, JOHN. *Fasti ecclesiae Anglicanae, 1300-1541. Vol.4: Monastic cathedrals (southern province)*, comp. B. Jones. Athlone Press, 1963.

For Gloucestershire clergy ordained in Exeter diocese, see:

S. W. 'Gloucestershire entries in Exeter episcopal registers', *G.N.Q.* **8**, 1901, 11-13. From Bishop Stafford's register, 1395-1419.

Lists of Gloucestershire abbots are provided by:

'The abbeys of Gloucestershire', *G.N.Q.* **7**, 1900, 105-10.

A number of works provide information concerning Gloucestershire clergy in the centuries immediately following the creation of the Diocese of Gloucester. These are arranged chronologically:

GAIRDNER, JAMES, ed. 'Bishop Hooper's visitation of Gloucester diocese, 1551', *English historical review* **19**, 1904, 98-121. Transcript of visitation return; gives names of clergy.

BASKERVILLE, G. 'Elections to convocation in the Diocese of Gloucester under Bishop Hooper', *English historical review* **44**, 1929, 1-32. Includes biographical notes on clergy named in the returns of 1552-3.

H., J.M. 'Married Gloucestershire clergy, 1554', *G.N.Q.* **3**, 1887, 42-3. List of those deprived under Mary.

FIELD, COLIN WALTER. *The state of the church in Gloucestershire, 1563*. Robertsbridge, Sussex: the author, 1971. Churchwardens' presentments, giving many names.

SHEILS, W.J., ed. 'A survey of the Diocese of Gloucester, 1603', in *An ecclesiastical miscellany*. B.G.A.S. Records Section **11**. Bristol: the Society, 1976, 59-102 and 145-51. Includes names of incumbents *etc*.

'Military assessment on the Gloucestershire clergy', *G.N.Q.* **5**, 1894, 126-31. In 1613, with names.

Religious Records continued

'The Gloucestershire ministers' testimony, 1648', *G.N.Q.* **1**, 1881, 329-31. Includes many ministers' signatures.

'Parliamentary survey of church livings, 1649-50: Co. Gloucester', *G.N.Q.* **2**, 1884, 214-22. Includes names of ministers *etc.*

ELRINGTON, C.R. 'The survey of church livings in Gloucestershire, 1650', *B.G.A.S.Tr.* **83**, 1964, 85-98. Includes names of many clergy.

Many histories of particular churches have been compiled, and frequently include clergy lists, the names of churchwardens, monumental inscriptions, parish register extracts *etc.* These cannot be listed here: you should ask one of the libraries listed on page 5 what is available. Lists of clergy in particular churches, together with other miscellaneous information, are provided by:

Arlingham
RAVENHILL, THOMAS HOLMES. 'Further particulars of Arlingham parish', *G.N.Q.* **2**, 1884, 74-7. Includes list of incumbents *etc.*

Ashleworth
'Ashleworth: ecclesiastical records', *B.G.A.S.Tr.* **48**, 1926, 275-86. Brief notes on deeds, wills, institutions, licences, tithes *etc.*

Bibury
BROWNE, A.L. 'The peculiar jurisdiction of Bibury', *B.G.A.S.Tr.* **58**, 1936, 171-95. Includes extracts from the Act Book, 1639, giving names.

Brimpsfield
BUTLER, RUTH F. 'Brimpsfield church history', *B.G.A.S.Tr.* **81**, 1962, 73-97. Includes biographical notes on incumbents.

Bristol
ATCHLEY, E.G.C.F. 'Documents relating to the parish church of All Saints, Bristol', *Archeological journal* **58**, 1901, 147-81. Various deeds and documents, including the will of Alice Halye, 1261.

ATCHLEY, E.G. CUTHBERT. 'On the medieval parish records of the church of St.Nicholas, Bristol', *Transactions of the St. Paul's Ecclesiological Society* **6**, 1906, 35-67.

FLETCHER, REGINALD JAMES. *A history of Bristol Cathedral, gathered from documents in the possession of the Dean and Chapter.* S.P.C.K., 1932. Includes list of members of the chapter.

Bristol *continued*

HOOPER, J. GRAHAM. 'The organs and organists of St. James, Bristol', *Organ* **28**(110), 1948, 75-82. Includes list, 1719-1940, with brief biographical notes.

JEAYES, J.H. 'Abbot Newland: roll of the abbots of St. Augustine's Abbey, Bristol', *B.G.A.S.Tr.* **14**, 1889-90, 117-30.

MASTERS, BETTY R. & RALPH, ELIZABETH, ed. *The church book of St.Ewen's, Bristol, 1454-1584.* B.G.A.S. Records Section **6**. Bristol: the Society, 1967. Includes churchwardens' accounts, lists of benefactors, deeds *etc.*

ORME, N.I. 'The Guild of Kalendars, Bristol', *B.G.A.S.Tr.* **96**, 1978, 32-49. Includes lists of priors and chaplains, 14-16th c.

WEARE, G.E. *A collectanea relating to the Bristol Friars Minor (Grey Friars) and their convent, together with a concise history of the dissolution of the houses of the four orders of mendicant friars in Bristol.* Bristol: W. Bennett, 1893. Gives names of some friars and benefactors.

A Guide to St. Mary Redcliffe church, Bristol; with a list of vicars, chaplains, etc., also biographical sketches of Canynges, Chatterton, etc. ... Bristol: C.T. Jefferies, 1858.

Brookthorpe
HALL, J. MELLAND. 'Some account of the parish of Brookthorpe', *B.G.A.S.Tr.* **13**, 1888-9, 359-83. Includes list of vicars, and lay subsidies, 1327 and 1557-8.

Charlton Kings
WYLLMER. 'Gloucestershire parish churches, III: St. Mary's, Charlton Kings', *G.N.Q.* **7**, 1900, 99-105. Includes lists of vicars, 1530-1783, and churchwardens, 1604-82.

'Ministers and incumbents at St. Mary's', *C.K.L.H.S.B.* **16**, 1986, 43-54. See also **17**, 1987, 48. List, with biographical notes.

Cirencester
See Winchcombe.

Coates
THORP, JOHN DISNEY. 'Rectors of Cotes or Coates', *B.G.A.S.Tr.* **48**, 1926, 301-24.

Condicote
WADLEY, THOMAS. 'Pre-Reformation incumbents of Condicote', *G.N.Q.* **4**, 1890, 391-2.

ROYCE, DAVID. 'Post-Reformation incumbents of Condicote', *G.N.Q.* **4**, 1890, 418-20.

Deerhurst
See Tewkesbury.

Religious Records continued

Gloucester

BRITTON, JOHN. *The history and antiquities of the Abbey, and Cathedral church of Gloucester, with biographical anecdotes of eminent persons connected with the establishment.* Longman, Rees, Orme, Brown, & Green, 1829. Includes lists of clergy, notes on monumental inscriptions *etc*.

ELLIS, MAY HEANE. 'The bridges of Gloucester and the hospital between the bridges', *B.G.A.S.Tr.* **51**, 1929, 169-210. Includes list of priors of St.Bartholomew's, Gloucester.

MEDLAND, HENRY. 'St. Oswald's Priory, Gloucester', *B.G.A.S.Tr.* **13**, 1888-9, 118-29. Includes list of priors.

'Chronological list of the abbots, and the buildings recorded to have been erected by them', *Records of Gloucester Cathedral* **2**, 1883-4, 174-6. *i.e.* of Gloucester Abbey.

Harescombe

'The rectors of Harescombe and Pitchcombe', *G.N.Q.* **2**, 1884, 288-90.

Hayles

See Winchcombe.

Hill

JENNER-FUST, H. 'The vicars of Hill parish, 1566-1887', *G.N.Q.* **3**, 1887, 594-6.

Icomb

W., A. 'Icomb parish: list of rectors', *G.N.Q.* **3**, 1887, 338-9.

Lantony

BADDELEY, W. ST. CLAIR. 'The story of the two Lantonys', *B.G.A.S.Tr.* **25**, 1902, 212-29. Includes list of priors.

LANGSTON, J.N. 'Priors of Lanthony by Gloucester', *B.G.A.S.Tr.* **63**, 1942, 1-143.

Lasborough

P., A.H. 'Lasborough parish: a list of rectors, etc.', *G.N.Q.* **3**, 1887, 645-7.

Nether Swell

ROYCE, DAVID. 'The church of St. Mary, Nether Swell', *B.G.A.S.Tr.* **7**, 1882-3, 45-55. Includes list of vicars.

Newland

MACLEAN, SIR JOHN. 'Notes on the Greyndour Chapel and Chantry in the church of Newland, Co. Gloucester, and on certain monumental brasses there', *B.G.A.S.Tr.* **6**, 1882-3, 117-25. Includes list of 15-16th c. chaplains.

Newnham

KERR, JOAN. 'Newnham parish magazine', *Local history bulletin* **40**, 1979, 9-11. Notes on an unusual source.

North Nibley

BUCKTON, J.D. 'The North Nibley tithe terrier', *B.G.A.S.Tr.* **41**, 1919, 205-22. 1619 list of tithepayers.

POPPLEWELL, JOYCE. 'A seating plan for North Nibley church in 1629', *B.G.A.S.Tr.* **103**, 1985, 179-84.

Nympsfield

SYMONDS, W. 'Brief notes on Nympsfield rectory', *G.N.Q.* **5**, 1894, 361-5. Includes list of rectors.

Pebworth

WADLEY, THOMAS PROCTER. 'Some particulars of the parish of Pebworth, Gloucestershire', *B.G.A.S.Tr.* **4**, 1879-80, 214-34. Includes list of incumbents, some lay subsidy rolls and extracts from the parish register.

Pitchcombe

See Harescombe.

Rendcombe

'Rendcombe church', *G.N.Q.* **10**, 1905, 33-41. Includes list of contributors to the relief of French protestants, 1686 *etc.*

Stratton on the Fosse

CORSE, S.E., & CAINE, J.M. 'Rectors of Stratton-on-the-Fosse, 1312-1930', *Downside review* **64**, 1946, 105-9, and **65**, 1947, 227.

Swell, Nether

See Nether Swell.

Tewkesbury

BICKERTON HUDSON, C.H. 'The Founders' book of Tewkesbury Abbey', *B.G.A.S.Tr.* **33**, 1910, 60-66. Notes on a manuscript giving biographical information on founders and patrons.

MASSE, H.J.L.J. *The abbey church of Tewkesbury, with some account of the priory church of Deerhurst, Gloucestershire.* George Bell & Sons, 1900. Includes list of Tewkesbury abbots, with notes on memorials.

ANTIQUARIUS. 'Tewkesbury Abbey and the pew system', *G.N.Q.* **2**, 1884, 57-9. Notes concerning the right to pews, 18th c.

Religious Records continued

Uley
PHILLIMORE, W.P.W. 'The rectors of Uley', *G.N.Q.* **2**, 1884, 162-8. See also 399-401.

Westbury on Trym
TAYLOR, C.S. 'The church and monastery of Westbury on Trym', *Proceedings of the Clifton Antiquarian Club* **4**, 1897-9, 20-42. Includes list of deans.

WILKINS, H.J. *Some chapters in the ecclesiastical history of Westbury on Trym ... to which is appended a list of abbots, deans and vicars since A.D.715.* Bristol: J.W.Arrowsmith, 1909.

WILKINS, H.J. *Westbury College from 1194 to 1544 A.D. ...* Bristol: J.W.Arrowsmith, 1917. Includes lists of deans, prebendaries *etc*.

Winchcombe
WALCOTT, MACKENZIE E.C. 'The abbeys of Winchcombe, Hayles, Cirencester, and Hales Owen', *Journal of the British Archaeological Association* **34**, 1878, 333-47. Includes lists of Gloucestershire abbots (Halesowen is in Worcestershire).

Denominations
Many denominations have been active in Gloucestershire, and especially in Bristol. Works of value to genealogists are listed below:

Huguenots
MAYO, RONALD. *The Huguenots in Bristol.* Local history pamphlets **61**. Bristol: Historical Association, Bristol Branch, 1985. Includes list of Huguenot refugees, giving places of origin.

LILLINGSTON, E.B.C. 'Bristol huguenots', *Proceedings of the Huguenot Society of London* **17**(3), 1944, 267-8. Brief note.

Methodists
KENT, JOHN. 'Wesleyan membership in Bristol, 1783', in *An ecclesiastical miscellany*. B.G.A.S. Record Section **11**. Bristol: the Society, 1976, 103-32 and 152-9. John Wesley's register of 790 members.

PILKINGTON, FREDERICK. 'Old King Street chapel, Bristol: an historic minute book', *Wesley Historical Society proceedings* **29**(6), 1954, 124-30. Description of minute book, 1794-1856.

Presbyterians and Baptists
STANLEY, JOHN. *In days of old: memories of the ejected ministers of 1662, their work and influence in the shires of Gloucester and Hereford.* Hereford: Herefordshire Press, 1913. Brief notes on many ministers.

Denominations:
Presbyterians *continued*

MURCH, JEROME. *A history of the Presbyterian and General Baptist churches in the West of England, with memoirs of some of their pastors.* R.Hunter, 1835. Includes list of ministers in Gloucestershire, Wiltshire, Somerset, Dorset, Devon and Cornwall.

HAYDEN, ROGER, ed. *The records of a church of Christ in Bristol, 1640-1687.* Bristol Record Society publications **27**. Bristol: the Society, 1974. Includes biographical notes, and supersedes previous editions by Underhill and Haycroft.

Quakers
TOWNSEND, JOHN. 'Some Gloucestershire quakers', *J.G.F.H.S.* **41**, 1989, 9-10. General discussion of sources, with list of Cirencester surnames.

MORTIMER, RUSSELL. *Early Bristol Quakers: the Society of Friends in the city, 1654-1700.* Bristol: Historical Association, Bristol Branch, 1967. Includes notes on archives of the Bristol Meeting.

MORTIMER, RUSSELL, ed. *Minute book of the Men's Meeting of the Society of Friends in Bristol, [1667-1704].* Bristol Record Society publications, **26** and **30**. Bristol: the Society, 1971-77. Includes biographical notes on persons mentioned.

Roman Catholics
Gloucestershire & North Avon Catholic History Society journal. Cheltenham: the Society, 1986-. Originally entitled *Newsletter*.

OLIVER, GEORGE. *Collections illustrating the history of the Catholic religion in the counties of Cornwall, Devon, Dorset, Somerset, Wilts. and Gloucester, in two parts: historical and biographical; with notices of the Dominican, Benedictine and Franciscan orders in England.* C. Dolman, 1857.

CLUTTERBUCK, R.H. 'State papers respecting Bishop Cheney, and the recusants of the diocese of Gloucester', *B.G.A.S.Tr.* **5**, 1880-1, 222-37. Includes petition of Bristol protestants, with names, 1568; list of Papists, 1577 *etc*.

KING, W.L. 'Gloucestershire recusants, 1715', *G.N.Q.* **2**, 1884, 101-3. List.

CRISP, H. & FERRY, V. 'Some Catholic families of Gloucestershire in the 18th c.', *Gloucestershire historical studies* **1**, 1966-7, 11-15.

HARDING, J.A. *Tercentenary of the Western District: Vicars Apostolic, Bishops of Clifton.* Bath: L.S.U. Publications, 1988. Mainly brief biographical notes on bishops.

Religious records: Denominations continued

Roman Catholics *continued*

HARDING, J.A. 'Vicars Apostolic of the Western District', *Gloucestershire & North Avon Catholic History Society journal* **6**, 1988, 6-13. Includes biographical notes.

BARTON, RICHARD. 'Missioners apostolic and rectors of Cheltenham', *Journal of the Gloucestershire & North Avon Catholic History Society* **14**, 1990, 33-4. List.

Swedenborgians

LEWIN, RON. 'New Jerusalem church', *J.B.A.* **31**, 1983, 1820. List of names appearing in church records, 1791-1968, including baptisms, marriages, roll *etc.*, of Bristol's Swedenborgian church.

Jews

ADLER, MICHAEL. 'The Jews of medieval Bristol', in his *Jews of medieval England*. Edward Goldston, 1939, 175-251. Includes list, 12th-13th c.

14. ESTATE AND FAMILY PAPERS

A. *GENERAL*

The records of estate administration (deeds, leases, rentals, surveys, accounts *etc.*) are a mine of information for the genealogist. Many of these records have been published in full or part, although far more still lie untouched in the archives. Few general collections of deeds have been published; for 'feet of fines' (*i.e.* medieval deeds), however, see:

MACLEAN, SIR JOHN. 'Pedes finium, or, excerpts from the feet of fines for the county of Gloucester from the 7th John [1205] to the 57th Henry III [1272]', *B.G.A.S.Tr.*, **16**, 1891-2, 183-95.

MACLEAN, SIR JOHN. 'Pedes finium, or, excerpts from the feet of fines, in the county of Gloucester, from the 30th Elizabeth [1587] to the 9th James I [1612]', *B.G.A.S.Tr.* **17**, 1892-3, 126-259.

'Extracts from Gloucestershire feet of fines', *G.N.Q.* **3**, 1887, 309-11, 325-8, 376-8 and 422-4. Index of names.

Other published notes on Gloucestershire deeds include:

L..J. 'Some genealogical notes', *G.N.Q.* **4**, 1890, 144-55. Gloucestershire extracts from a *Calendar of Privy Seals, signed bills, etc. (Chancery series),* covering the years 1625-36, and mainly concerned with conveyancing.

'Gloucestershire charters', *Archaeological journal* **29**, 1872, 268-72. See also **28**, 1871, 159-60. Medieval deeds.

From deeds and other manorial documents it is usually possible to trace the descent of manors. Many descents are given in:

ROBINSON, W.J. *West country manors*. Bristol: St. Stephens Press, 1930.

See also:

COOKE, ROBERT. *West Country houses: an illustrated account of some country houses and their owners in the counties of Bristol, Gloucester, Somerset and Wiltshire, being also a guide to domestic architecture from the reign of Henry II to Victoria.* Batsford, 1957. Includes notes on the descent of the houses described.

KINGSLEY, NICHOLAS. *The country houses of Gloucestershire.* Cheltenham: the author, 1989. Includes brief notes on owners *etc.*

Estate Papers: General continued

The process of enclosing land from open field resulted in the creation of many documents. Enclosure awards usually include complete lists of owners and tenants, and are consequently invaluable for genealogists. Awards for Gloucestershire are listed in:

TATE, W.E. 'Gloucestershire enclosure acts and awards', *B.G.A.S.Tr.* **64**, 1943, 1-70.

Early insurance policy registers represent an important, if under-used, genealogical source. For Bristol, see:

REDSTONE, A. 'Insurance policy registers as source material for the genealogist', *J.B.A.* **1**, 1975, 25-32, and **2**, 1975, 17-25. Includes alphabetical listing of policy holders, early 18th c.

B. PRIVATE ESTATES

Many families have preserved deeds and papers relating to their estates. A number of these have been published and are listed here.

Blaythwayt

SMITH, BRIAN S. 'Blathwayt of Dyrham Park archives', *Archives* **5**(28), 1962, 224-5. Brief note on family papers, 17-18th c.

Fitzhardinge

JEAYES, ISAAC HERBERT. *Descriptive catalogue of the charters and muniments in the possession of Lord Fitzhardinge at Berkeley Castle*. Bristol: C.T. Jefferies & Son, 1892.

Gloucester, Earldom of

PATTERSON, ROBERT B., ed. *Earldom of Gloucester charters: the charters and scribes of the Earls and Countesses of Gloucester to A.D.1217*. Oxford: Clarendon Press, 1973.

Hatton Wood

TAYLOR, F. 'The Hatton Wood manuscripts in the John Rylands Library', *Bulletin of the John Rylands Library* **24**, 1940, 353-75. Brief description of a collection which, although primarily of Cheshire interest, does include charters from Kent, Gloucestershire *etc*.

Hereford, Earldom of

WALKER, DAVID, ed. 'Charters of the Earldom of Hereford, 1095-1201', in *Camden miscellany* **22**. Camden 4th series **1**. Royal Historical Society, 1-75. See also index, 179-94. Gloucester family charters, including many relating to Gloucestershire. See also: WALKER, DAVID. 'The "Honours" of the Earls of Hereford in the twelfth century', *B.G.A.S.Tr.* **79**(2), 1960, 174-211.

Neale

NEALE, J.A. *Charters and records of Neales of Berkeley, Yate and Corsham*. Warrington: Mackie & Co., 1907. See also supplement, 1927, and further addenda, 1929. Mainly relating to Wiltshire and Gloucestershire.

Sherborne, Barons of

A calendar of the charters, rolls, and other documents (dating from 1182) as contained in the muniment room at Sherborne House, in Gloucestershire, belonging to the Right Honourable the Lord Sherborne, Baron of Sherborne. [ ]: privately printed, 1900. Relating to many Gloucestershire manors, especially Sherborne and Bibury, and to the families of Dalton and Stawell.

Estate Papers: Private continued

Shrewsbury, Earls of
SCROGGS, EDITH S. 'The Shrewsbury (Talbot) manuscripts: Gloucestershire references', *B.G.A.S.Tr.* **60**, 1938, 26-96. Deeds *etc*.

Smith
MILLER, CELIA, ed. *The account books of Thomas Smith, Irley Farm, Hailes, Gloucestershire, 1865-71*. B.G.A.S. Records Section **13**. Bristol: the Society, 1985. Includes many names.

Smythe
VANES, JEAN, ed. *The ledger of John Smythe, 1538-1550*. Bristol Record Society **28**. Bristol: the Society, 1975. Also published in Historical Manuscripts Commission joint publications series **19**. H.M.S.O., 1975. Includes pedigree.

Spillman
WATSON, C.E. 'The Spillman Cartulary', *B.G.A.S.Tr.* **61**, 1939, 50-94. Spillman family deeds; includes notes on Spillman and Payne families, medieval.

Many estate records relating to particular places are in print, and are listed here by locality:

Abinghall
See Dene Magna.

Achards
See Stonehouse.

Alveston
'Manor of Alveston', *G.N.Q.* **3**, 1887, 293-6. Medieval descent of manor.

Ashley
See Cheltenham.

Aston Subedge
M., J. 'The manor of Aston sub Edge', *G.N.Q.* **1**, 1881, 140-42. See also 164-5. 17th c. descent of manor.

Badminton
'Gloucestershire farmers and high prices of corn, 1795', *G.N.Q.* **2**, 1884, 54-5. Agreement by tenants of the Duke of Beaufort's Badminton estate, giving names.

Berkeley Hundred
'Berkeley Hundred court rolls', *G.N.Q.* **5**, 1884, 85-88. Transcript of roll for 1543.

Birts Morton
MACLEAN, SIR JOHN. 'Notes on the manors and advowsons of Birts Morton and Pendock', *B.G.A.S.Tr.* **10**, 1885-6, 186-225. Descent of the manors, with list of rectors and patrons, and pedigrees of Nanfan.

Bitton
ELLACOMBE, H.T. *The history of the parish of Bitton, in the county of Gloucester*. Exeter: William Pollard, 1881. Includes court rolls, inquisitions post mortem, subsidies, pedigrees *etc*.

ELLACOMBE, H.T. 'Some account of the manor of Button or Bitton, Co. Gloucester', *Herald & Genealogist* **4**, 1867, 193-212 and 311-20. Includes descent of manor.

GOULSTONE, JOHN. 'Some early deeds for Bitton', *J.B.A.* **52**, 1988, 35-6. 16-17th c. deed abstracts in the library of the Society of Genealogists.

Bristol
BICKLEY, FRANCIS B., ed. *Calendar of deeds (chiefly relating to Bristol) collected by George Weare Braikenridge*. Edinburgh: T. & A. Constable, 1899. Mainly medieval.

BIRCH, WALTER DE GRAY. 'Original documents relating to Bristol and the neighbourhood', *Journal of the British Archaeological Association* **31**, 1875, 289-305. Includes medieval deeds, 1445 rental *etc*. See 516-8 for index.

WAY, LEWIS JOHN UPTON. 'Some miscellaneous Bristol deeds', *B.G.A.S.Tr.* **42**, 1920, 97-123.

'Ancient Bristol documents', *Proceedings of the Clifton Antiquarian Club* **1**, 1884-8, 51-7, 136-55; **2**, 1888-93, 152-6 and 244-56; **3**, 1893-6, 25-34, 151-61 and 228-34; **4**, 1897-9, 12-16 and 109-38; **5**, 1900-3, 205-9; **6**, 1904-8, 180-91 and 216-21; **7**, 1909-12, 46-50 and 83-5. Includes notes on many deeds, records of losses in the civil war at Westbury upon Trym and Clifton, will of Stephen le Spicer, 1337/8 *etc*.

BIRCH, WALTER DE GRAY. 'Original documents relating to Bristol and the neighbourhood', *British Archaeological Association journal* **31**, 1875, 289-305. Deeds, 1125-1505.

HARDING, N. DERMOTT, ed. *Bristol charters, 1155-1373*. Bristol Record Society publications **1**. Bristol: the Society, 1930.

HICKS, F.W. POTTO 'Original documents of the thirteenth century relating to Bristol', *B.G.A.S.Tr.* **58**, 1936, 219-42. Deeds.

CRONNE, H.A., ed. *Bristol charters, 1378-1499*. Bristol Record Society publications **11**. Bristol: the Society, 1946.

Estate Papers: Private continued

Bristol *continued*

BADDELEY, ST. CLAIR. 'A Bristol rental, 1498-9', *B.G.A.S.Tr.* **47**, 1925, 123-9.

LATHAM, R.C., ed. *Bristol charters, 1509-1899.* Bristol Record Society publications **12**. Bristol: the Society, 1946.

RALPH, E. 'Grants and leases of lands in King Street, Bristol', *B.G.A.S.Tr.* **65**, 1944, 160-66. Mainly a list of 1663 leases.

FRANCE, R. SHARPE, [ed.]. 'An 18c. Bristol rental', *Notes & Queries* **178**, 1940, 78. Of lands belonging to the parish of Christ Church, 1725.

Brockworth

BARTLEET, S.E. 'History of the manor and advowson of Brockworth', *B.G.A.S.Tr.* **7**, 1882-3, 131-71. Includes pedigree of Chandos, 12-13th c., list of vicars, and notes on many deeds *etc.*

Chalfield
See Great Chalfield.

Chalford

RUDD, MARY A. 'Abstracts of deeds relating to Chalford and Colcombe', *B.G.A.S.Tr.* **51**, 1929, 211-24.

Charlton Kings

GREET, M.J. 'Some medieval deeds of the 14th and 15th c.', *C.K.L.H.S.B.* **13**, 1985, 4-7. Tabulated information from Charlton Kings' deeds.

PAGET, MARY. 'Charlton in 1617, taken from the extent of the manor of Cheltenham ...', *C.K.L.H.S.B.* **18**, 1987, 35-40.

PAGET, MARY. 'A rental of Cheltenham manor about 1450: the Charlton section (G.R.O. D. 855 M. 68)', *C.K.L.H.S.B.* **15**, 1986, 10-18. Charlton Kings.

WELCH, F.B. 'The manor of Charlton Kings, later Ashley', *B.G.A.S.Tr.* **54**, 1932, 145-65. Includes descent of the manor.

Cheltenham

PAGET, MARY. 'A study of manorial custom before 1625', *Local historian* **15**, 1982, 166-73. Inheritance customs *etc.*, on the manors of Cheltenham and Ashley.

Chipping Campden

BARNARD, E.A.B. 'Court books of the borough of Chipping Campden, 1769-1886', *Evesham notes & queries* **2**, 1911, 175-82.

Clifford Chambers

MACLEAN, SIR JOHN. 'History of the manor and advowson of Clifford Chambers, and some account of its possessors', *B.G.A.S.Tr.* **14**, 1889-90, 50-99. Includes extent, 1266, descent of the manor, pedigree of Rainsford, 15-17th c., list of rectors *etc.*

Clifton

ELLIS, ALFRED S. 'On the manorial history of Clifton', *B.G.A.S.Tr.* **3**, 1878-9, 211-29. Manorial descent to 17th c.

LATIMER, JOHN. 'Clifton in 1746', *B.G.A.S.Tr.* **23**, 1900, 312-22. Map, with list of occupants. See also: LATIMER, JOHN. 'Clifton in 1746', *Proceedings of the Clifton Antiquarian Club* **5**, 1900-3, 25-34.

WAY, LEWIS J. UPTON. 'The 1625 survey of the smaller manor of Clifton', *B.G.A.S.Tr.* **36**, 1913, 220-50.

See also Bristol.

Coates

THORP, JOHN DISNEY. 'History of the manor of Coates, County Gloucester', *B.G.A.S.Tr.* **50**, 1928, 135-274. Includes descent of the manor, with pedigree of Poole, Atkyns, Tombs, Dewe, *etc.*

Colcombe
See Chalford.

Cold Ashton

BUSH, THOS. S. 'Records of Cold Ashton', *G.N.Q.* **9**, 1902, 40, 85-9, 129-37, and 175-77. Court rolls, lay subsidy *etc.*, 14-15th c.

Dene Magna

MACLEAN, SIR JOHN. 'The history of the manors of Dene Magna and Abenhall and their Lords; also fugitive notes on the manors of Parva Dene, Ruardyn and Westbury', *B.G.A.S.Tr.* **6**, 1881-2, 123-209. Includes lists of rectors, pedigrees of Dene, Abenhall, Baynham, Greyndour, Vaughan, Roberts, Colchester and Probyn; rental of *c*.1519 *etc.*

Dowdeswell

HILL, MARY C. 'Dowdeswell Court Book, 1577-1673', *B.G.A.S.Tr.* **67**, 1946-8, 119-216. See also **68**, 1949, 202.

Estate Papers: Private continued

English Bicknor
MACLEAN, SIR JOHN. 'Court roll of the manor of Bicknor Anglicana, Co. Gloucester', *B.G.A.S.Tr.* **11**, 1886-7, 269-79. 1638.

MACLEAN, SIR JOHN. 'Remarks on the manor, advowson, and demesne lands of English Bicknor, Co. Gloucester', *B.G.A.S.Tr.* **1**, 1876, 69-95. Descent of manor, including pedigrees of Wyrall, 14-19th c., and of Muchegros, Ferrers and Devereux, 13-17th c., with list of rectors, and subsidy of 1522/3.

Filton
CLEVERDON, S. 'The manor and advowson of Filton', *Notes on Bristol history* **5**, 1962, 57-61. Descent of the manor, 1580-1832.

Flaxley Grange
HEANE, W.C. 'Flaxley Grange', *B.G.A.S.Tr.* **6**, 1881-2, 284-305. Descent of the property, including pedigrees of Kingston, Brayne, Hawkins, and Skippe, 16-19th c.

Gloucester
WALKER, DAVID. 'Ralph, son of Richard', *Bulletin of the Institute of Historical Research* **33**(88), 1960, 194-202. Deeds relating to tenements in Gloucester, 12th c.

STEVENSON, W.H. ed. *Rental of all the houses in Gloucester, 1435, from a roll in the possession of the Corporation of Gloucester.* Gloucester: John Bellows, 1890.

Great Chalfield
DAVIES, J. SILVESTER. 'The manor and church of Great Chalfield', *B.G.A.S.Tr.* **23**, 1900, 193-261. Includes descent of the manor, pedigrees of Tropenell, Percy, and Eyre, list of patrons and incumbents of Great and Little Chalfield *etc.*

Hanham
'Hanham court', *G.N.Q.* **6**, 1896, 143-9. Descent of the manor.

Henbury
WAY, LEWIS J. UPTON. 'The owners of the Great House, Henbury, Gloucestershire', *B.G.A.S.Tr.* **33**, 1910, 304-37. Descent of the house.

Huntley
EASTWOOD, J.M. 'The Huntley manor estate 1717-1883', *Gloucestershire historical studies* **8**, 1977, 34-40. General discussion based on estate documents, with many names, and including notes on Probyn family.

Kempley
BADDELEY, W. ST. CLAIR. 'The history of Kempley manor and church, Gloucestershire', *B.G.A.S.Tr.* **36**, 1913, 130-51. Descent of the manor, including pedigrees of De Miners, 12-14th c., and De Longchamp, 12-13th c., with list of clergy.

King's Stanley
See Stonehouse.

Little Chalfield
See Great Chalfield.

Little Rissington
BROWNE, A.L. 'The early lords of Little Rissingdon', *B.G.A.S.Tr.* **53**, 1931, 219-35. Descent of the lordship.

Minchinhampton
WATSON, C. ERNEST. 'The Minchinhampton custumal and its place in the story of the manor', *B.G.A.S.Tr.* **54**, 1932, 203. Includes names of many medieval tenants.

Miserden
BADDELEY, ST. CLAIR, W. 'Miserden and its owners', *Proceedings of the Cotteswold Naturalists' Field Club* **20**, 1918-20, 45-58. Descent of manor, with pedigree of Sandys, 16-18th c.

Parva Dene
See Dene Magna.

Pauntley
CONDER, EDWARD. 'Pauntley manor and the Pauntley custom', *B.G.A.S.Tr.* **40**, 1917, 115-31. Includes descent of the manor, with pedigree of Whittington and Poole, 14-17th c.

Pendock
See Birts Morton.

Pitchcombe
HALL, JOHN MELLARD. 'Pychenecumbe: abstracts of original documents in the registers of the Abbey of St. Peters, Gloucester', *B.G.A.S.Tr.* **14**, 1889-90, 141-62. Charters.

Prestbury
BROWNE, A.L. 'Title deeds of the manor of Prestbury, Gloucestershire', *B.G.A.S.Tr.* **61**, 1939, 281-6. 16-17th c.

Estate Papers: Private continued

Prinknash
BASELEY, WILLIAM. 'History of Prinknash Park', *B.G.A.S.Tr.* **7**, 1882-3, 267-306. Includes pedigrees of Brydges, 15-17th c., Bray, 14-16th c., Seymour, 14-16th c., and Bridgeman, 15-18th c.
LEOTARD, ALBAN. 'Families connected with the history of Prinknash', *J.G.F.H.S.* **8**, 1981, 14-15. Includes brief descent of manor.

Rissington, Little
See Little Rissington.

Ruardyn
See Dene Magna.

Southam
HUDDLESTON, C. ROY. 'The builder of Southam and some deeds connected with the estate', *B.G.A.S.Tr.* **50**, 1928, 275-311. Includes descent of the estate, with will of Sir John Huddleston, 1545, deed extracts *etc.*
'Some ancient deeds relating to the manor of Southam, near Cheltenham', *B.G.A.S.Tr.* **28**, 1905, 48-60. Includes pedigrees of Huddlestone, Delabere, and Baghot.

Staunton
MACLEAN, SIR JOHN. 'History of the manor and advowson of Staunton, in the Forest of Dean', *B.G.A.S.Tr.* **7**, 1882-3, 227-66. Includes pedigrees of Hall and Gage, 16-19th c., *inquisitions post mortem* for Thomas Staunton, 1476 and John Staunton, 1526; rental, 1584-5, and list of rectors *etc.*

Stonehouse
SWYNNERTON, CHARLES. 'Some early court rolls of the manors of Stonehouse, Kings Stanley, Woodchester and Achards', *B.G.A.S.Tr.* **45**, 1923, 203-52. 15-17th c. rolls.

Tetbury
WALKER, T. WARBURTON. 'Some notes on Tetbury, its church and court leet', *B.G.A.S.Tr.* **37**, 1914, 61-78. Includes survey of 1594, listing tenants.

Thornbury
H., R.A.G. 'Records of an English manor for a thousand years', *Genealogical magazine* **4**, 1901, 377-83 and 425-31.

Tockington
MACLEAN, SIR JOHN. 'Manor of Tockington, Co. Gloucester, and the Roman villa', *B.G.A.S.Tr.* **12**, 1887-8, 123-69, and **13**, 1888-9, 247-51. Includes descent of the manor, pedigree of Poyntz, 11-17th c., and Berkeley, 14-16th c., list of medieval incumbents *etc.*

Upton St. Leonard's
RUFFELL, JOHN V. 'The court rolls of Upton St. Leonard's', *Local history bulletin* **48**, 1983, 3-5. 16th c.
SCOBELL, E.C. 'The common fields at Upton Saint Leonards and the recent inclosure (1897)', *Proceedings of the Cotteswold Naturalists' Field Club* **13**, 1899-1901, 215-30. Includes list of landowners from 1840 tithe apportionment.

Walton Cardiff
DOWDESWELL, E.R. 'Some ancient deeds illustrating the devolution of an estate in the manor of Walton Cardiff, near Tewkesbury, between the years A.D.1166 and 1833', *B.G.A.S.Tr.* **32**, 1909, 165-76.

Wanswell Court
COOKE, JAMES HERBERT. 'Wanswell Court and its occupants for seven centuries', *B.G.A.S.Tr.* **6**, 1881-2, 310-23. Descent of the property, including pedigrees of Stone, Swanhunger and Thorpe, 13-17th c., and Lysons, 17-19th c.

Westbury on Severn
See Dene Magna.

Westbury on Trym
See Bristol.

Woodchester
See Stonehouse.

Estate Papers continued

C. ECCLESIASTICAL ESTATES AND CARTULARIES, ETC.

In the medieval period, a great deal of property was owned by ecclesiastical institutions such as churches, monasteries, dioceses *etc*. Ecclesiastical estate records have survived much better than those of private families, and many are in print. The 'terriers' of the diocese of Gloucester, which provide information on property owned by churches, are listed in:

Gloucester diocese terriers. Local history pamphlets **4**. Gloucester: Gloucester City Libraries, 1964.

Printed records of particular ecclesiastical bodies include:

Bristol
All Hallows
NICHOLLS, J.F. 'Old deeds of All Hallows Church, Bristol', *Journal of the British Archaeological Association* **31**, 1875, 259-65.

St. Augustine's
BEACHCROFT, GWEN, & SABIN, ARTHUR, eds. *Two compotus rolls of St. Augustine's Abbey, Bristol, for 1491-2 and 1511-12*. Bristol Record Society publications **9**. Bristol Record Society, 1938. Includes list of canons *etc*.

SABIN, ARTHUR, ed. *Some manorial accounts of St. Augustine's Abbey, Bristol, being the computa of the manors for 1491-2 and 1496-7 and other documents of the fifteenth and sixteenth centuries*. Bristol Record Society publications **22**. Bristol: the Society, 1960.

St. Mark's Hospital
ROSS, C.D. ed. *Cartulary of St. Mark's Hospital, Bristol*. Bristol Record Society publications **21**. Bristol: the Society, 1959. Includes notes on some 13th c. mayors and bailiffs.

St. Nicholas
WAY, LEWIS J. UPTON. 'The early charters of Saint Nicholas Church, Bristol', *B.G.A.S.Tr.* **44**, 1922, 121-44. 12-14th c.

Cirencester Abbey
ROSS, C.D., & DEVINE, MARY, eds. *The chartulary of Cirencester Abbey, Gloucestershire*. 3 vols. Oxford University Press, 1964-77.

Flaxley
CRAWLEY-BOEVEY, ARTHUR W., ed. *Cartulary and historical notes of the Cistercian Abbey of Flaxley, otherwise called Dene Abbey, in the county of Gloucester*. Exeter: W. Pollard & Co., 1887.

Gloucester
The major source relating to St. Peter's Abbey is:
HART, WILLIAM HARRY, ed. *Historia et cartularium monasterii S. Petri Gloucestriae*. 3 vols. Rolls series **33**. Longman, Green, Longman, Roberts & Green, 1863-7. **1-2** includes numerous 12-13th c. deeds; **3** has manorial extents, 1265-7 and various judicial records. See also:

BADDELEY, W. ST. CLAIR. 'Early deeds relating to St. Peter's Abbey, Gloucester', *B.G.A.S.Tr.* **37**, 1914, 221-34, and **38**, 1915, 19-46. See also **38**, 1915, 47-68.

HILTON, R.H. 'Gloucester Abbey leases of the late 13th century', *University of Birmingham Historical journal* **4**(1), 1953, 1-17. General discussion of the cartulary.

WALKER, DAVID. 'A register of the churches of the monastery of St. Peter's, Gloucester', in *An ecclesiastical miscellany*. B.G.A.S. Record Section **11**. Bristol: the Society, 1976, 1-58 and 133-44. Medieval chartulary.

WALKER, DAVID. 'Some charters relating to St. Peter's Abbey, Gloucester', *in* BARNES, PATRICIA M., & SLADE, C.F., eds. *A medieval miscellany for Doris Mary Stenton*. Pipe Roll Society, N.S. **36**. The Society, 1960, 247-68. 12-13th c.

Kingswood
LINDLEY, E.S. 'A Kingswood Abbey Rental', *B.G.A.S.Tr.*, **70**, 1951, 145-51. 1445; includes many names.

PERKINS, V.R. 'Documents relating to the Cistercian monastery of St. Mary, Kingswood', *B.G.A.S.Tr.* **22**, 1899, 179-256.

Llanthony
JACK, R. IAN. 'An archival case history: the cartularies and registers of Llanthony Priory in Gloucestershire', *Journal of the Society of Archivists* **4**, 1970-73, 370-83. General discussion of the Priory's archives.

Winchcombe
ROYCE, DAVID, ed. *Landboc. Sive registrum monasterii beatae Mariae Virginis et Sancti Cenhelmi de Winchelcumba ...* 2 vols. Exeter: William Pollard, 1892-1903. Includes many 13-16th c. deeds. See also: P. 'List of charters in the Winchcombe cartularies, in the possession of Lord Sherborne', *Collectanea topographica et genealogica* **2**, 1835, 16-39.

15. NATIONAL, COUNTY AND LOCAL ADMINISTRATION

A. NATIONAL AND COUNTY

Official lists of names, such as tax lists and census schedules, have already been discussed. There are, however, many other records of central and local government which provide useful information. For general background information on governmental activities in Gloucestershire and Bristol, see:

WILLCOX, WILLIAM BRADFORD. *Gloucestershire: a study in local government, 1590-1640.* New Haven: Yale University Press, 1940.

MOIR, ESTHER. *Local government in Gloucestershire, 1775-1800: a study of the justices of the peace.* B.G.A.S. Records Section **8**. Bristol: the Society, 1969. Includes a list of J.P's.

RALPH, ELIZABETH. *The government of Bristol, 1373-1973.* Bristol: Corporation of Bristol, 1973. Brief general history of local government.

Most of Gloucestershire's leading families have sent a member to represent the county or a local borough in parliament. Biographical information on them is contained in:

WILLIAMS, W.R. *Parliamentary history of the county of Gloucester, including the cities of Bristol and Gloucester, and the boroughs of Cheltenham, Stroud and Tewkesbury, from the earliest times to the present day, 1213-1898, with biographical and genealogical notices of the members.* Hereford: Jakeman & Carver for the author, 1898. This is continued by: HYETT, SIR FRANCES, & WELLS, CHARLES. 'Members of Parliament for Gloucestershire and Bristol, 1900-29', *B.G.A.S.Tr.* **51**, 1929, 321-60. See also: DRIVER, J.T. 'Parliamentary Burgesses for Bristol and Gloucester, 1422-1437', *B.G.A.S.Tr.* **74**, 1955, 60-127.

See also *English genealogy: an introductory bibliography,* chapter 12, D.

National and county administration has produced a wide range of documents of interest to genealogists, some of which have been published, and are listed here chronologically:

MAITLAND, F.W., ed. *Pleas of the Crown for the county of Gloucester before the Abbot of Reading and his fellow justices itinerant ...1221.* Macmillan, 1884.

STENTON, DORIS MARY, ed. *Rolls of the justices in eyre, being the rolls of pleas and assizes for Gloucestershire, Warwickshire, and Staffordshire, 1221, 1222.* Selden Society **59**. The Society, 1940.

WATSON, EDWARD JAMES. *Pleas of the Crown for the hundred of Swineshead and the township of Bristol ... 1221.* Bristol: W. Crofton Hemmons, 1902.

WELCH, F.B. 'Gloucestershire in the Pipe Rolls', *B.G.A.S.Tr.* **57**, 1935, 49-109, and **59**, 1937, 185-209. Accounts rendered by the sheriff to the crown in the 12th c., recording many names.

BARKLY, SIR HENRY. 'A Gloucestershire jury list of the thirteenth century', *B.G.A.S.Tr.* **10**, 1885-6, 293-303.

KIMBALL, ELIZABETH GUERNSEY, ed. *Rolls of the Gloucestershire sessions of the peace, 1361-1398.* Issued as *B.G.A.S.Tr.* **62**, 1940.

S., A.B. 'Gloucestershire justices of the peace', *G.N.Q.* **5**, 1894, 142-6. Lists for 1483, 1485, 1509, 1547, 1553 and 1670.

GRAY, IRVINE. 'A Gloucestershire postscript to the "Domesday of inclosures"', *B.G.A.S.Tr.* **97**, 1979, 75-80. Returns for Gloucestershire, 1517, giving names of jurors and landowners *etc.*

MACLEAN, SIR JOHN. 'On feudal and compulsory knighthood', *B.G.A.S.Tr.* **9**, 1884-5, 345-53. Includes list of Gloucestershire men fined for not taking the order of knighthood in 1625.

'Dring's catalogue of compounders, 1655', *G.N.Q.* **1**, 1881, 374-6. List of royalists fined for their loyalty.

'Gloucestershire address to King Charles II, 1660', *G.N.Q.* **1**, 1881, 165-7. Address of welcome, with many signatures of the leading gentry.

MACLEAN, SIR JOHN. 'Seizure of arms in the county of Gloucester in 1684', *B.G.A.S.Tr.* **2**, 1877-8, 104-17. Lists supporters of the Duke of Monmouth from whom arms were seized.

BROWNE, A.L. 'Penal laws in Gloucestershire', *B.G.A.S.Tr.* **61**, 1939, 287-93. Lists deputy lieutenants and justices of the peace, giving their reputed opinions on toleration, in response to an inquiry by James II.

GLOUCESTRENSIS. 'The sheriffs of Gloucestershire, 1779-1886', *G.N.Q.*, 3, 1887, 414-7. List.

SMITH, BRIAN S. 'Sheriffs of Gloucestershire since 1832', *B.G.A.S.Tr.* **86**, 1967, 183-92. List.

EVERETT, DAVID. 'Gloucestershire inquests', *J.G.F.H.S.* **41**, 1989, 7-8. 1790-92.

Local Administration continued

The charities in the County of Gloucester: selected from the voluminous reports of the Commissioners for Inquiry concerning Charities in England and Wales, which began the 58th year of the reign of Geo.III [1817] and ended the 7th of Will.IV. [1837] James Newman, 1839. See also *G.N.Q.* **2**, 1884, 417-25. For Bristol, see: MANCHEE, THOMAS JOHN, ed. *Bristol charities, being the report of the Commissioners for inquiring concerning charities in England and Wales, so far as relates to the charitable institutions in Bristol.* 2 vols. Bristol: the editor, 1831.

B. PAROCHIAL AND CITY ADMINISTRATION

The records of parochial government – the accounts of overseers, churchwardens, and other parish officers, settlement papers, rate lists *etc.* – contain much information of genealogical value. They frequently provide the names, if nothing else, of the humble mass of the poor, who otherwise went unrecorded. Surviving Gloucestershire records are listed in:
GRAY, IRVINE & RALPH, ELIZABETH, eds. *Guide to the parish records of the city of Bristol and the county of Gloucester.* B.G.A.S. Records Section **5**. Bristol: the Society, 1963.

Many extracts from municipal, parochial, and family accounts, giving names, may be found in:
DOUGLAS, AUDREY & GREENFIELD, PETER, eds. *Cumberland, Westmorland, Gloucestershire. Records of early English drama.* Toronto: University of Toronto Press, 1986.

Many Gloucestershire folk were subjected to settlement examination in other counties. Some from Wolverley, Worcestershire, are given in:
EVERETT, DAVID M. 'Settlement examinations: Wolverley, Worcestershire', *J.G.F.H.S.* **23**, 1984, 5-8. See also **24**, 1985, 24.

Gloucestershire and Bristol municipal and parochial records have been the subject of many books and articles. Some of those likely to be of genealogical interest are listed here:

Bedminster
PHILLIPS, JUDITH. 'Poor relief in Bedminster, 1833', *J.B.A.* **2**, 1975, 13-16 and **3**, 1976, 20-3; **4**, 1976, 1620. List of persons claiming relief.

Berkeley
See Hinton.

Bisley
H., 'Bisley churchwarden's account, 1630', *G.N.Q.* **2**, 1884, 482. Includes names.

Bitton
WYALL, IRENE & JOHN. 'The poor law records of Bitton', *Gloucestershire historical studies* **5**, 1972, 31-44. See also **6**, 1974-5, 35-4. General discussion with some names.

Brislington
AUSTIN, A. 'Brislington parish church: churchwardens' accounts, 1681-1730', *J.B.A.* **41**, 1985, 37-9. General description.

Administration: Parochial and City continued

Bristol

This list is arranged in rough chronological order, with parochial records at the end.

BEAVEN, ALFRED B. *Bristol lists: municipal and miscellaneous*. Bristol: T.D. Taylor, Sons, & Hawkins, 1899. Lists of mayors, aldermen, and numerous officers *etc.*, with brief biographical notes. See also: BEAVEN, A.B. *The municipal representation of Bristol (1835-1880)*. Bristol: the author, 1880, for lists of M.P's, J.P's, and various other officers.

HARDING, N. DERMOTT. 'The archives of the Corporation of Bristol', *B.G.A.S.Tr.* **48**, 1926, 227-49.

HUDD, ALFRED E. 'Two Bristol calendars', *B.G.A.S.Tr.* **19**, 1894-5, 105-41. List of medieval mayors, sheriffs, bailiffs *etc.*

RICART, ROBERT. *The Maire of Bristowe is kalendar*, ed. Lucy Toulmin Smith. Camden Society, N.S. **5**. The Society, 1872. Includes names of medieval mayors, bailiffs, etc. See also: LATIMER, JOHN. 'The Maire of Bristowe is Kalendar: its list of civic officers collated with contemporary legal mss', *B.G.A.S.Tr.* **26**, 1903, 108-37.

BICKLEY, FRANCIS B., ed. *Little red book of Bristol*. 2 vols. Bristol: W. Crofton Hemmons; London: Henry Sotheran & Co., 1900. Medieval.

VEALE, E.W.W., ed. *The great red book of Bristol*. Bristol Record Society publications, **2**, **4**, **8**, **16** and **18**. Bristol: the Society, 1931-53. Includes many deeds, with full calendar of feet of fines, 12-14th c., also some wills, rentals, letters *etc.*

FULLER, E.A. 'Pleas of the Crown at Bristol, 15 Edward I [1286-7]', *B.G.A.S.Tr.* **22**, 1899, 150-78. Includes list of 33 wine sellers.

CARUS-WILSON, E.M., ed. *The overseas trade of Bristol in the later middle ages*. Bristol Record Society publications **7**. Bristol: the Society, 1937. Includes list of enrolled customs and subsidy accounts, list of mayors and constables of the staple, 1354-71, and pedigree of Canynges, 15th c.

RALPH, ELIZABETH, ed. *The great white book of Bristol*. Bristol Record Society publications **32**. Bristol: the Society, 1979. 16th c. custumal, giving many names.

RICH, E.E., ed. *The staple court books of Bristol*. Bristol Record Society publications **5**. Bristol: the Society, 1934. 16th c. court cases; many names.

LIVOCK, D.M., ed. *City chamberlains' accounts in the sixteenth and seventeenth centuries*. Bristol Record Society publications **24**. Bristol: the Society, 1966.

BRISTOL RECORD OFFICE. *Records of poor law administration*. Information leaflet **5**. Bristol: the Office, 1985. Brief pamphlet.

PITT, W. PEPPERELL. 'The coroners of Bristol', *B.G.A.S.Tr.* **55**, 1933, 135-41. List, 17-19th c.

NOTT, H.E. & RALPH, ELIZABETH, eds. *The deposition books of Bristol*. Bristol Record Society publications **6** and **13**. Bristol: the Society, 1935-48. Transcripts of sworn statements made before the mayor and aldermen, with biographical notes on mayors and officers *etc.*, 1643-54.

BUTCHER, E.E., ed. *Bristol Corporation of the Poor: selected records, 1696-1834*. Bristol Record Society publications **3**. Bristol: the Society, 1932.

BUTCHER, E.E. *Bristol Corporation of the Poor: 1696-1898*. Local history pamphlets **29**. Bristol: Historical Association, Bristol Branch, 1972. General discussion.

RALPH, ELIZABETH & McGRATH, PATRICK, eds. *Records of Bristol quarter sessions for the eighteenth century*. Notes on Bristol history **9**. Bristol: University of Bristol Dept. of Extra-Mural Studies, 1971. Transcripts.

LAMOINE, GEORGES, ed. *Bristol gaol delivery fiats, 1741-1799*. Bristol Record Society publications **40**. Bristol: the Society, 1989.

'A list of persons killed and wounded at the Bristol riots, 30 September 1793', *J.B.A.* **29**, 1982, 32-33.

BUSH, GRAHAM. *Bristol and its municipal government, 1820-1851*. Bristol Record Society publications **29**. Bristol: the Society, 1976. Includes biographical notes on members of the Corporation and town councillors.

NEALE, W.G. *At the Port of Bristol*. 2 vols. Bristol: Port of Bristol Authority, 1968. Includes biographical notices of members of the Bristol Docks Committee, 1848-1914.

All Saints

ATCHLEY, E.G. CUTHBERT F. 'On the parish records of All Saints, Bristol', *B.G.A.S.Tr.* **27**, 1904, 221-74. General discussion; includes list of rectors to 1600.

St. Ewens

MACLEAN, SIR JOHN. 'Notes on the accounts of the procurators, or churchwardens, of the parish of St. Ewen's, Bristol', *B.G.A.S.Tr.* **15**, 1890-91, 139-82 and 254-96. 15th c. transcript.

Administration: Parochial and City continued

Campden
POWELL, GEOFFREY. 'Shovelling out the Campden paupers', *Local history bulletin* **52**, 1985, 13-17. 19th c., includes extracts from churchwardens' accounts.

Charlton Kings
GREET, M.J. 'Charlton Kings parish workhouse, 1826-1836', *C.K.L.H.S.B.* **3**, 1980, 42-50. Includes list of inmates.

Cheltenham
GRAY, IRVINE, ed. *Cheltenham settlement examinations, 1815-1826*. B.G.A.S. Records Section **7**. Bristol: the Society, 1969.

Childs Wickham
SMITH, GEORGE. 'Childswickham memorandum book, 1755-1799', *Evesham notes & queries* **2**, 1911, 190-9.

Cirencester
S., E.C. 'Bond of inhabitants of Cirencester for prosecution of felons, 1774', *G.N.Q.* **3**, 1887, 158-60. Signatures of 162 inhabitants.

Coln St. Dennis
MUNN, K.M. 'The accounts of the overseers of the poor of Coln St. Dennis, 1776-1812', in SMITH, BRIAN S., ed. *Gloucestershire historical studies* **1**, 1966-7, 16-21.

Eastington
ABHBA. 'Extracts from the accounts of the churchwardens of Eastington, 1616-1756', *G.N.Q.* **3**, 1887, 246-54.

Forest of Dean
HART, CYRIL E. *The commoners of Dean Forest*. Gloucester: British Publishing Co., 1951. Includes extensive list of claimants at Eyre of the Forest, 1634.

HART, CYRIL E. *The free miners of the royal Forest of Dean and hundred of St. Briavels*. Gloucester: British Publishing Co., 1953. Includes many names of jurors *etc.*

HART, CYRIL E., ed. *The regard of the Forest of Dene in 1282: translation, comments, notes.* [ ]: Forest of Dean Local History Society, 1987. In effect a survey of the Forest; many names.

HART, CYRIL E. *The verderers and forest laws of Dean*. Newton Abbot: David & Charles, 1971. Includes list of Forest officials, 1282, with many other names.

Gloucester
FRYER, KEDGWIN HOSKINS. 'The archives of the city of Gloucester', *B.G.A.S.Tr.* **1**, 1876, 59-68.

STEVENSON, WILLIAM H. *Calendar of the records of the Corporation of Gloucester*. Gloucester: John Bellows, 1893. There is an mss supplement to this calendar edited by V.A. Woodman at Gloucester City Library.

STEVENSON, W.H., ed. 'The records of the Corporation of Gloucester', in *The manuscripts of the Duke of Beaufort, K.G., the Earl of Donoughmore, and others*. Historical Manuscripts Commission, 12th report, appendix, pt.9. C.6338. H.M.S.O., 1891, 400-529.

Hampnett
WIGGIN, WILLIAM. 'The accounts of the churchwardens of Hampnett parish, 1607-19', *G.N.Q.*, **2**, 1894, 113-6. Includes names of churchwardens *etc*.

Hinton
HAINES, ROBERT J. 'The overseer of the poor book, Hinton, Berkeley', *J.G.F.H.S.* **39**, 1988, 26-8. See also **40**, 1989, 12. Brief extracts.

Iron Acton
STRANGE, A. 'Perambulations of Iron Acton parish in 1695 and 1745', *J.B.A.* **20**, 1980, 13. Lists of participants in the perambulations.

Matson
'Charles Gibbs, parish clerk of Matson, and his predecessors', *G.N.Q.* **3**, 1887, 37-41.

Minchinhampton
BRUCE, JOHN. 'Extracts from accounts of the churchwardens of Minchinhampton, in the county of Gloucester', *Archaeologia* **35**, 1854, 409-52.

Mitcheldean
The poor in Mitcheldean, 1660-1834. Bristol: University of Bristol Dept. of Extra-Mural Studies, 1962.

Northleach
ROYCE, DAVID. 'The Northleach court book', *B.G.A.S.Tr.* **7**, 1882-3, 90-116. Includes list of officers, 1547-1701, with many other names.

Sevenhampton
GLOUCESTRENSIS. 'Sevenhampton parish: churchwardens, 1616-1683', *G.N.Q.* **3**, 1887, 508-9. List.

Shirehampton
See Westbury on Trym.

Administration: Parochial and City continued

Stoke Bishop
See Westbury on Trym.

Stroud
'Stroud vestry minute book', *G.N.Q.* **5**, 1894, 69-71. Includes list of churchwardens, 1756-83.

Tetbury
'Landlords, tenants and owner occupiers in Tetbury, 1838', *History of Tetbury Society journal* **12**, 1987, 5-10. 1838 rate.

Welford
STORR, F. 'The petty constable's accounts of Welford on Avon, 1687-1735', *Gloucestershire historical studies* **6**, 1974-5, 16-22. General discussion; includes some names.

Westbury on Trym
'A private collection of Westbury archives', *J.B.A.* **18**, 1979, 20-21. Parochial records of Westbury-on-Trym.

WILKINS, H.J., ed. *Transcriptions of the 'poor book' of the tithings of Westbury on Trym, Stoke Bishop, and Shirehampton, from A.D.1656-1698, with introduction and notes.* Bristol: J.W. Arrowsmith, 1910. Accounts, including many lists of taxpayers.

Weston sub Edge
ASHBEE, C.R. *The last records of a Cotswold community: being the Weston Subedge field account book for the final twenty-six years of the famous Cotswold Games ...* Chipping Camden: Essex House Press, 1904. Includes accounts, 1826-52, of open field administration, giving many names.

16. EDUCATION

The records of schools can provide the genealogist with a great deal of information. For the history of Gloucestershire schools in the medieval period, see:

ORME, NICHOLAS. *Education in the West of England, 1066-1548: Cornwall, Devon, Dorset, Gloucestershire, Somerset, Wiltshire.* Exeter: University of Exeter, 1976.

There are many histories of individual schools, and a few school registers have been published. School histories usually list headmasters; they may also include the names of assistant teachers and/or pupils. Some, of course, are of much more genealogical value than others. The following list is not comprehensive; rather, it seeks to identify those school histories which possess some genealogical value.

Bristol
MORGAN, EDWIN THOMAS. *A history of the Bristol Cathedral School.* Bristol: J.W. Arrowsmith, 1913. Includes brief list of headmasters.

SAMPSON, WALTER ADAM. *History of Queen Elizabeth's Hospital, Bristol.* Bristol: John Wright & Sons, 1910. This 'Hospital' is in fact a school. Includes list of masters, with a chapter on 'John Carr and his will'. The will was dated 1574.

SAMPSON, WALTER ADAM. *A history of the Bristol Grammar School.* Bristol: J.W. Arrowsmith, 1912. Includes various lists of masters and scholars *etc*.

Charlton Kings
MIDDLETON, H. 'The log book of Higgs' night school, 1877-1896' (G.R.O. P76 SC 4/2), *C.K.L.H.S.B.* **20**, 1988, 30-33. Charlton Kings.

Cheltenham
BELL, ARTHUR. *Tudor foundation: a sketch of the history of Richard Pate's foundation in Cheltenham.* Chalfont St. Giles: Richard Sadler for the Pate Foundation, 1974. Includes list of schoolmasters 1574-1971, and detailed references to sources.

PIGG, CHARLES HERBERT, ed. *Cheltenham College register, 1841-1919; additions and corrections, 1919-1951.* Cheltenham: the College, 1953.

Cheltonian honours list, 1841-1900. Cheltenham: John Darter, [c.1900]. List of academic honours won by Cheltenham College students at the universities *etc*.

Education continued

Clifton
BEACHCROFT, S.P., ed. *Clifton College register, 1862 to 1962*. Bristol: J.W. Arrowsmith for the Old Cliftonian Society, 1962.
EVANS, J.S. *Clifton College register, 1962-1978*. Clifton: the College, 1979.

Gloucester
LEPPER, CHARLES. *The Crypt School, 1539-1989: the story of the Crypt School, Gloucester, seen through the eyes of its pupils and teachers during its first 450 years*. Gloucester: Alan Sutton, 1989. Includes extensive 'index of people named'.
ROBERTSON, DAVID. *The King's School, Gloucester*. Chichester: Phillimore, 1974. Includes list of sources with many names listed in index, and list of masters and ushers, 16-20th c.
LANGSTON, J.N. 'Headmasters and ushers of the King's (College) School, Gloucester, 1541-1841', *Records of Gloucester Cathedral* **3**, 1885-1927, 148-236. Biographical notes. For index (to whole journal) see 237-44.
The Kings School, Gloucester, otherwise known as the College School. Gloucester: Mirchim & Gibbs, 1912. Includes register of old boys with addresses.

Kingswood
HASTLING, A.H.L., et al. *The history of Kingswood School, together with registers of Kingswood School and Woodhouse Grove School, and a list of masters*. Charles H. Kelly, 1898. See also:
HASTLING, A.H.L., ed. *Register of Kingswood School*. 3rd.ed. Brentford: [ ], 1923. The school moved to Bath, in Somerset, 1851.

Wotton under Edge
HORNSBY, F.W.D., & GRIFFIN, K. *Katherine, Lady Berkeley's School, Wotton under Edge, 1384-1984*. Wotton: the School, 1984. Many names noted in index; includes detailed list of sources.

Wycliffe
WARD, R.V. *A register of old Wycliffians, 1882-1937*. Gloucester: John Bellows, 1937.

17. EMIGRATION

Gloucestershire place-names are frequently found in countries far removed from their origin. One thinks of Randwick Airport in New South Wales, of Gloucester, Massachusetts (and also in New South Wales), of no less than six Bristols to be found in the United States. These places were all founded by Gloucestershire men and women. But how to trace them? It is not the purpose here to list everything published on Gloucestershire emigrants, but rather to indicate a few of the works readily available in England which may be useful. Further assistance may be had by consulting the works listed in Chapter 16 of *English genealogy: an introductory bibliography*.

Australia
The most useful work, based on Gloucestershire quarter sessions records, is:
WYATT, IRENE, ed. *Transportees from Gloucestershire to Australia, 1783-1842*. Gloucestershire record series **1**. Gloucester: B.G.A.S., 1988. See also: AMEY, G. *City under fire, the Bristol riots and aftermath*. Guildford: Lutterworth Press, 1979. Includes biographical notices of convicts transported to Australia in 1831.
CLUTTERBUCK, JERRY. 'A list of 42 convicts from Gloucester, tried in Gloucester and sent to Australia on the first fleet', *J.G.F.H.S.* **35**, 1987, 18.
DUNCAN, R. 'Case studies in emigration: Cornwall, Gloucestershire, and New South Wales', *Economic history review*, 2nd series **16**(2), 1963, 272-89.

South Africa
WILLIAMS, J. ROBERT. 'Gloucestershire settlers in the Eastern Cape', *J.G.F.H.S.* **16**, 1983, 8-10. Includes list of emigrants in 1820.

United States of America
COLDHAM, PETER WILSON. *The Bristol registers of servants sent to foreign plantations, 1654-1686*. Baltimore: Genealogical Publishing, 1988. Records 10,000 emigrants mainly from the West Country, Wales and the West Midlands, who passed through Bristol.
HARGREAVES-MAWDSLEY, R. 'Bristol records: a representative list of persons who emigrated to America between the years 1654 and 1679', *Apollo* **6**, 1927, 29-31.

FAMILY NAME INDEX

Abenhall 66
Adams 53, 54
Adeane 24
Africanus 54
Agg 20
Alye 20
Annesley 20
Apsley 20
Archard 20
Arnolde 44
Arrowsmith 20
Arundel 44
Arundell 20, 46
Astry 23
Atkyns 20, 66
Avenel 20
Baghot 68
Barclay 20
Barnard 20
Barnes 20
Barrow 20, 29
Bartlett 20
Bathe 44
Bathurst 20
Batten 20
Baynham 66
Beaufort 65
Beaufort, Dukes of 73
Berewe 29
Berkeley 11, 20, 21, 53, 68
Biddill 46
Bigland 21
Birche 45
Birt 45
Blagden 25
Blake 47
Blathwayt 64
Booth 20
Boteler 30
Bovey 53
Bower 21
Bradeston 21
Bradwey 45
Bray 21, 53, 68
Brayne 67
Bridgeman 68
Britton 21

Broadway 45
Brooke 21
Brown 22
Browne 22
Browning 46
Brydges 22, 68
Bubb 22
Buckingham, Dukes of 29
Budgett 22
Burcombe 45
Busby 22
Bushell 22
Butler 27, 45
Camber 45
Cambray 22
Canning 22
Canynges 22, 60, 71
Capel 45
Carr 74
Carruthers 27
Cary 22, 27
Cassey 22
Catchmay 22
Challoner 27
Chandos 22, 66
Chatterton 22, 60
Chester 23
Clare 23
Cleeveley 23
Clifford 23
Clopton 53
Clutterbuck 23, 45
Coates 29
Codrington 23, 53
Colchester 23, 66
Collet 23
Cornock 53
Cotton 20
Cowmeadow 23
Creswicke 45
Crossman 23
Crupes 29
Currier 20
Dadswell 23
Dalton 64
Daston 45
Daubeney 23

Daubrie 23
Daunsey 46
Daunt 23
Davies 24, 29
De Chedder 24
De Havilland 24
De Longchamp 67
De Miners 24, 67
Deane 24
Deen 45
Deighton 24
Delabere 68
Dene 24, 66
Devereux 67
Dewe 66
Dimock 24
Diston 45
Dixton 44, 45
Dobell 24
Dorney 24
Dowdeswell 24
Dudbridge 24
Dutton 24
Dymer 32
Eden 24
Edgeworth 24
Edwards 24
Elton 28
Elyce 45
Eyre 67
Ferrers 67
Finnimore 24
Fitzhardinge 64
Forster 24
Fortescue 24
Foster 53
Fowler 25, 53
Fox 25
Freeman 25, 28, 53
French 47
Fust 25
Gage 68
Gale 45
Garlick 25
Garnes 25
Gayner 25
Gibbes 25

Family Name Index

Gibbs 73
Giffard 25, 45
Gifford 23
Gloucester 64
Gloucester, Earls of 64
Gookin 23, 25
Gorges 27
Gostlett 26
Gough 25
Grace 25
Graile 53
Graves 25
Green 25
Gregory 54
Grevill 25
Greville 25
Greyndour 61, 66
Guise 25
Hale 25
Hall 68
Hallewell 25
Halye 60
Hamlett 26
Harding 21
Harington 26
Hart 45, 47
Hartland 26
Harvey 45
Hatton Wood 64
Havelland 23
Haviland 23
Hawkins 67
Hawthorne 26
Haynes 26
Heane 26
Hearne 28
Heavens 45
Hereford, Earls of 64
Hicks 26
Hicks Beach 26
Hillier 26
Hine 27
Hodges 26, 45
Holbrow 26, 53
Holder 21
Hooke 26
Hopkins 26
Horton 45
Howard 29
Huddleston 68
Huddlestone 68
Hungerford 26
Huntington 45

Hutchens 46
Hutchyns 30, 31
Jacobs 26
Jenkinson 26, 53
Jenner 21, 27
Jennings 27
Jerningham 27
Johnson 27
Jones 28, 53
Jordan 27
Kelke 53
Kent 27
Kerr 27
Kingscote 21, 27
Kingston 67
Knatchbull 22
Knight 27
Lane 27
Langley 27, 45
Latch 27
Lawrence 27, 29
Leigh 27
Little 27
Lond 53
Longden 27
Longe 28
Looge 45
Loud 53
Loveday 40
Ludlow 28
Lyde 53
Lyne 28, 46
Lynett 46
Lysons 28, 68
Mace 28
Machen 28
Makeig 28
Marisall 28
Marshall 28, 46
Martin 28
Martyn 28
Matthews 28
Mayo 28
Merrett 53
Merryweather 46
Michell 46
Miles 46
Mitchell 53
Monoux 28
Moore 28
Morgan 46
Morton 46
Muchegros 67

Muchgros 28
Muir 53
Myll 46
Nanfan 65
Neale 64
Newland 53, 60
Oldisworth 28
Oliver 28
Osborne 28
Overbury 28-9, 46
Palling 27
Parker 29
Parkin 29
Parry 26
Parsons 27
Partridge 53
Paston 29
Pate 74
Paul 7, 29, 53
Paulet 29
Pauncefote 29
Pawlett 29
Payne 46, 65
Percy 67
Pettat 53
Phelps 29
Phillipps 29
Pillinger 29
Poole 66, 67
Pope 29
Porter 53
Pouldon 53
Poulton 46
Poyntz 29, 68
Probyn 26, 66, 67
Prowde 46
Pynke 46
Rainsford 66
Randwick 24
Redcle 46
Robert 21
Roberts 66
Robin 29
Robins 54
Robinson 29
Rodway 46
Rogers 46
Rooke 29
Rowlands 29
Rudder 29
Russell 29
Rutter 46
Saintloe 54

Family Name Index

Sandys 67
Sargeaunt 29
Sargent 29
Sawnders 46
Scrope 26
Scrupes 30
Seager 28
Selk 46
Selwyn 30
Semys 54
Seymour 68
Sheppard 30
Sherborne 24, 64, 69
Shipton 46
Shipway 29
Shrewsbury, Earls of 65
Skippe 67
Slaughter 29
Sly 54
Smith 46, 65
Smyth 10, 11, 21, 29
Smythe 46, 65
Snigge 54
Somers 46
Sowle 46
Spicer 65
Spillman 65
Stafford 29, 47
Staunton 68
Stawell 64

Stephens 29
Stiff 30
Stokes 30
Stone 68
Stonehouse 24
Stradlynge 47
Stratford 54
Sturge 30
Sturmy 47
Sudeley 30
Swanhunger 68
Talbot 65
Tame 25, 31, 50
Teague 31
Terrill 23
Thorpe 68
Throckmorton 31
Tippett 31
Todeni 31
Tombs 31, 66
Tomes 31, 45
Tracy 31
Trevisa 48
Tropenell 67
Trotman 31
Twining 30
Tyler 30
Tyndale 20, 30, 31
Vaughan 66
Wakeham 47

Walcot 31
Walter 46
Ware 47
Washbourne 31
Watkins 45
Watts 47
Wayte 47
Weight 31
White 27, 47
Whitefield 32
Whitmore 53
Whitson 32
Whittington 32, 47, 67
Willets 32
Willett 32
Williams 32, 47
Wills 32, 54
Wilson 54
Winston 54
Wood 32, 54
Woodroffe 32
Woodward 54
Wynter 32
Wyntour 32
Wyrall 32, 67
Wytloff 47
Yeend 32
Yescombe 32
Yonge 31, 54
Young 26, 32, 54

PLACE NAME INDEX

Bedfordshire 23
Berkshire: Reading 20
Cambridgeshire: Cambridge 58
Cheshire 57, 64
    Dutton 24
Co. Durham: Selaby 28
Cornwall 13, 18, 44, 62, 74, 75
Cotswolds 7 12, 13, 21, 25, 26, 31, 57
Cumberland 71
Derbyshire 34
Devon 13, 18, 62, 74
    Exeter Diocese 59
    Ladyswill 47
    Plymouth 36
    Stonehouse 36
Dorset 13, 18, 24, 28, 43, 62, 74
    Long Barton 54
    Wyke Regis 34
Essex: Walthamstow 20, 28
Gloucestershire and Bristol
    Abenhall 34, 66
    Abson 26
    Achards 68
    Acton Turville 35, 42
    Adlestrop 34
    Alderley 25, 35
    Alderton 34, 46
    Aldsworth 34
    Almondsbury 23, 35, 48
    Alveston 65
    Alvington 35
    Ampney 34
    Ampney Crucis 35
    Arlingham 35, 60
    Ashchurch 35
    Ashleworth 23, 28, 29, 34, 60
    Ashley 66
    Ashton under Hill 34
    Aston Blank 37
    Aston Somerville 34, 35
    Aston sub Edge 34, 35, 39 46, 65
    Avening 30, 35
    Badgeworth 48
    Badminton 65
    Badsey 39

Gloucestershire *continued*
    Badgeworth 48
    Badminton 65
    Badsey 39
    Bagendon 34
    Barnsley 34
    Barnwood 34
    Barton Regis 23
    Bartonbury 22
    Batsford 28, 34, 35
    Baunton 34
    Beckford 34
    Beckington 48
    Bedminster 25, 56-58, 71
    Berkeley 21, 35, 53, 57, 64, 73
    Berkeley Castle 19, 21, 48, 64
    Berkeley Hundred 11, 18, 21, 65
    Beverston 26, 35
    Bibury 34, 43, 60, 64
    Birts Morton 65
    Bishops Cleeve 34, 35, 43
    Bisley 17, 34, 48, 55, 71
    Bisley Hundred 7, 55
    Bitton 26, 35, 65, 71
        Upton Cheyney Manor,
        Upton House 29
    Blaisdon 34
    Bledington 34
    Boddington 34
    Bourton on the Hill 28, 34
    Bourton on the Water 27, 35
    Boxwell 35
    Bradley Hundred 17
    Bream. New Inn 25
    Brightwells Barrow Hundred 7
    Brimpsfield 23, 25, 34, 35, 60
    Brimpsfield Castle 25
    Brimscombe 48
    Brislington 25, 29, 71
    Bristol 7-26, 28-3,35, 36, 43-48, 53, 55-58, 62-66, 70-72, 75
        All Hallows 69
        All Saints 36, 46, 60, 72
        Arno's vale 49
        Brandon Hill, St. George's 36, 48, 49

Glos.: Bristol *continued*
    Castle precincts 56
    Christ Church 36, 48, 56, 66
    Council House 15
    Holy Trinity 36
    King Street 66
    Lawfords Gate Prison 15
    Mayor's Chapel 49
    Merchants Hall 15
    Old King Street Chapel 62
    Queen Elizabeth's Hospital 74
    Red Lodge 19, 32
    Redland Court 28
    St. Augustine the Less 36, 56
    St. Augustine's 60, 69
    St. Augustine's Back, Great House 27
    St. Ewen's 60, 72
    St. James 36, 60
    St. John the Baptist 36, 56
    St. Mark's 49
    St. Mark's Hospital 69
    St. Mary le Pont 36
    St. Mary Redcliffe 22, 36, 48, 56, 60
    St. Michael 36
    St. Nicholas 36, 48, 56, 60, 69
    St. Paul 36
    St. Peter 53
    St. Peter's Hospital 56
    SS. Philip & Jacob 36
    St. Philip's 36
    St. Stephen 36, 54, 56
    St. Thomas 36, 56
    St. Werbergh 36, 49
    Temple 36, 56
    Temple St. Sugar House 27
    Trenchard Lane, St.Joseph's Chapel 35
    Whitson Court Sugar House 29

Place Name Index

Gloucestershire *continued*
Bristol Cathedral 19, 36
  54, 60
Bristol Cathedral School 74
Bristol Deanery 49
Bristol Diocese 11, 33, 43
Bristol Grammar School 74
Britwells Barrow Hundred 17
Broad Marston 22
Broadwell 34, 36
Brockthorpe 46, 55
Brockworth 34, 49, 66
Bromsberrow 34, 36
Brookthorpe 36, 60
Buckland 34, 36
Bushley 25, 36, 53
Button 65
Cainscross 48, 49
Cam 30, 36, 55
Campden 15, 36, 73
Chalford 49, 66
Charlton Abbotts 34
Charlton Kings 12, 14, 17, 23,
  34, 36, 44, 49, 58, 60, 66,
  73, 74
  The Knappings 20
Chavenage 29
Chedworth 34, 36, 54
Cheltenham 12, 14, 17, 19,
  29, 34, 36, 48, 49, 55, 58,
  60, 66, 73, 74
  Christ Church 49
  St. James 49
  St. Mary's 49
  St. Peter's 49
  Trinity 49
Cheltenham College 74
Cheltenham Hundred 55
Cherington 34, 36
Childs Wickham 34, 36, 73
Chipping Campden 19, 49, 66
Chipping Campden Deanery
  49
Chipping Sodbury 28, 37, 49
Churchdown 34
Cirencester 26, 37, 44, 46,
  48, 50, 57, 62, 73
  St. John's 50
Cirencester Abbey 69
Cleeve Hundred 7
Clifford Chambers 34, 37, 66
Clifton 12, 29, 37, 44, 50, 57,
  58, 65, 66

Gloucestershire *continued*
Clifton College 75
Clifton Diocese 11, 62
Clingre 31
Clowerwall 31
Coaley 37
Coates 34, 51, 60, 66
Coberley 20, 34
Codrington 23, 42
Colcombe 66
Cold Ashton 32, 34, 37, 66
Colesbourne 30, 34
Coln Rogers 34, 37
Coln St.Aldwyn 34
Coln St.Dennis 34, 73
Compton Abdale 34
Condicote 34, 60
Coombe Hill 50
Corse 34
Cotes 60
Cowley 34
Cranham 34, 50, 55
Cricklade 57
Cromhall 50
Cubberley 50
Cutsdean 34
Daglingworth 34, 51
Deerhurst 34, 61
  Wightfield 22
Deerhurst Hundred 7
Dene Abbey 69
Dene Magna and Parva 66
Detmore 24
Didbrook 34
Didmarton 23
Dodington 21, 23, 37
Dorrington 34
Dorsington 37
Dowdeswell 34, 66
Down Hatherley 34
Doynton 37
Driffield 34, 51
Drystowe 47
Dumbleton 34, 45
Duntisbourne Abbots 37
Duntisbourne Rous 37
Dursley 20, 29, 30, 37, 50, 57
Dymock 19, 34, 37
Dyrham 37
Dyrham Park 64
Eastington 37, 45, 73
Eastleach Martin 34
Eastleach Turville 34
Ebrington 34, 37, 39

Gloucestershire *continued*
Edge 48
Edgeworth 34, 37
Elkstone 34, 37
Elmore 25, 55
Elmstone Hardwicke 34
English Bicknor 34, 66, 67
Evenlode 34
Eyford 42
Fairford 19, 31, 37, 50, 57
Farmcote 54
Farmington 34
Filton 37, 50, 67
Fishponds 50
Flaveley 53
Flaxley 34, 69
Flaxley Grange 67
Forest (North) Deanery 50
Forest of Dean 14, 31, 56, 58
  68, 73
Forthampton 34, 37
Frampton 17, 23
Frampton Cotterell 44
Frampton on Severn 23, 37
Frocester 38
Gloucester 7-11, 13, 18, 24,
  27, 44, 46, 53, 57, 58,
  67, 70, 73, 75
  Barton Street Chapel 38
  Christ Church 34
  Crypt School 75
  King's School 75
  St. Aldate 34
  St. Bartholomew 61
  St. John the Baptist 34, 54
  St. John's 38
  St. Mary de Crypt 34
  St. Michael's 34, 44
  St. Oswald's 61
  St. Peter's Abbey and
    Cathedral 11, 15, 50, 61
    67, 69
  Southgate Street Chapel 38
Gloucester Deanery 50
Gloucester Diocese 11, 33,
  43, 59, 62, 69
Great Badminton 38
Great Barrington 21, 34, 53
Great Chalfield 67
Great Rissington 22, 38
Great Washbourne 34
Great Witcombe 34, 50
Guiting Power 34, 38

Place Name Index

Gloucestershire *continued*
Guiting Temple 34
Hailes 34
Irley Farm 65
Hampnett 34, 38, 73
Hanham 38, 67
Hardwicke 38
Harescombe 38, 46, 50, 61
Haresfield 34, 45, 55
Harnhill 34
Hartpury 34
Hasfield 29, 34
Hatherop 38, 51
Hawkesbury 26, 30, 38, 53
Hawkesbury Deanery 50
Hawling 34
Hayles 62
Hazelton 34
Hempstead 34
Hempsted 53
Henbury 29, 38, 54
Henbury. Great House 67
Hewelsfield 24, 34
Hewletts 20
Highfield 25
Hill 25, 38, 50, 61
Hinton 73
Hinton on the Green 34, 38
Honeybourne 24
Horsley 38
Horton 21, 29, 38
Hotwells 57, 58
Huntley 38, 67
Icomb 22, 38, 61
Iron Acton 38, 45, 73
Kemerton 38
Kempley 19, 67
Kempsford 38
Kings Stanley 25, 39, 50, 68
Kingscote 21, 26, 27, 39
Kingsdown. Montague Street 57
Kingswood 16, 39, 50
Kingswood Abbey 69
Kingswood Chase 21
Kingswood Hill 22
Kingswood School 75
Langley Hundred 56
Lanthony 45, 61
Lasborough 61
Lassington 34, 53
Lechlade 20, 57
Leckhampton 50, 58
Leigh 45, 51
Leighterton 35

Gloucestershire *continued*
Lemington Parva 39
Leonard Stanley 23, 26, 39, 47, 51
Little Barrington 34
Little Chalfield 67
Little Compton 28, 34
Little Rissington 39. 67
Little Sodbury 45
Little Washbourne 31
Llanthony Priory 69
Long Marston 35, 39
Longhope 34
Longhope, Hart Barn 29
Longney 51
Longtree 17
Longtree Hundred 7, 55
Lower Slaughter 39
Maisemore 39, 51
Mangotsfield 44, 56
Marlwood 47
Marshfield 39
Marston Sicca 31, 39
Matson 35, 39, 73
Mickleton 25, 35, 39
Minchinhampton 30, 39, 67, 73
Minsterworth 39
Highgrove 20
Miserden 35, 51, 67
Mitcheldean 20, 35, 39, 73
Moreton 22
Moreton in Marsh 35, 39
Motson 30
Nailsworth 48
Naunton 35, 39
Nether Swell 39, 61
Newent 35
Newington Bagpath 39
Newland 26, 35, 61
Newnham 27, 61
Nibley 11, 29, 30, 46, 53
North Cerney 34, 51
North Nibley 40, 61
Northleach 35, 51, 57, 73
Northleach Deanery 51
Norton 35
Notgrove 35
Nympsfield 27, 40, 61
Oakridge 48, 51
Oddington 35
Old Sodbury 40
Oldbury on Severn 40
Oldbury on the Hill 40, 51
Oldland 38

Gloucestershire *continued*
Olveston 40, 42, 55, 56
Owlpen 40
Oxenhall 34
Oxenton 35
Ozleworth 40
Painswick 27, 32, 35, 40, 51, 53, 57
   Dell Farm, Friends' Burial Ground 40
Parva Dene 66
Pauntley 19, 34, 67
Pebworth 35, 40, 61
Pendock 65
Pitchcombe 35, 40, 46, 51, 61, 67
Plusterwine 31
Postlip 53
   St. James Chapel 51
Poulton 35
Prestbury 40, 51, 58, 67
   New Cemetery 49
Preston 35
Preston upon Stour 35, 40
Prinknash 68
Prinknash Park 68
Pucklechurch 40
Quedgeley 33, 40
Quenington 34
Quinton 34, 40, 53
Radgeworth 34
Ramsgate Hundred 7
Randwick 24, 34, 51
Redland 51, 58
Redland Green 51
Redmarley 34
Rendcombe 34, 40, 61
Rockhampton 51, 52
Rodborough 46, 52
Rodmarton 28, 34
Ruardean 34, 66
Rudford 34
Saint Briavels 24, 34, 47
Saint Briavels Hundred 73
Saintbury 34, 40
Salperton 34
Sandhurst 34
Sapperton 34, 51, 52
Sevenhampton 41, 73
Sheepscombe 48
Sherborne 24, 41, 64
Shipton Moyne 26, 41
Shipton Oliffe 45
Shirehampton 7, 52, 74

Place Name Index

Gloucestershire *continued*
Siston 41, 47
Slade 48
Slaughter Hundred 7
Slimbridge 41
Snowshill 41
South Cerney 34
Southam 68
Southrop 41
Standish 41, 54
Stanton 19, 41
Stanton Drew 53
Stanway House 19
Staunton 34, 68
Stinchcombe 26, 30, 41
Stoke Bishop 74
Stone 41
Stonehouse 25, 41, 52, 68
Stonehouse Deanery 52
Stow Deanery 52
Stowell 38
Stratton on the Fosse 61
Stroud 46, 52, 57, 58, 70, 74
   Rodborough Tabernacle 52
Sudeley 22, 30, 43
Swindon 41, 52
Swineshead Hundred 56, 70
Syde 41
Syston 30, 41
Taynton 21, 34
Temple Guiting 41
Tetbury 12, 41, 47, 57, 68, 74
Tewkesbury 15, 20, 28, 52, 57, 70
   Barton Street 52
   Holy Trinity 52
Tewkesbury Abbey 19, 52, 61
Tewkesbury Hundred 7
Thornbury 13, 29, 36, 42, 68
Tibberton 34
Tibblestone Hundred 7
Tidenham 42
Tirley 42
Tockington 68
Toddington 19, 31
Todenham 42
Tormarton 42
Tortworth 31, 42
Tredington 42
Turkdean 42, 52
Twining 42
Uley 21, 24, 26, 42, 45, 46, 55, 62

Gloucestershire *continued*
Upleadon 34
Upper Slaughter 42
Upton on Severn 13
Upton St.Leonards 34, 68
Walton Cardiff 34, 68
Wanswell Court 68
Wapley 42
Welford 34, 74
West Littleton 42
Westbury 44, 66
Westbury College 22
Westbury Hundred 7
Westbury on Trym 17, 26, 42, 51, 54, 62, 64, 74
Westcote 34, 42
Westminster Hundred 7
Weston Birt 7, 42
Weston Subedge 34, 39, 42, 74
Weston upon Avon 34
Whaddon 42
White Cross 32
Whitstone 17
Whitstone Hundred 7
Whittington 30, 34
Wick 26
Wickwar 42
Widford (now Oxon.) 34
Willersey 34, 42
Winchcombe 34, 43, 62, 69
Winchcombe Deanery 52
Windrush 26, 34, 43
Winson 34
Winstone 43
Winterbourne 19
Withington 34, 43
Withy Holt 27
Woodchester 22, 43, 52, 68
Woodhouse Grove School 74
Wotton under Edge 12, 31, 45, 52, 57, 75
Wyck Risington 43
Wycliffe School 75
Yarworth 34
Yate 21, 52, 64
Gloucestershire, North 17
Gloucestershire, South 16, 33, 34
Hampshire & Isle of Wight 18
Herefordshire 20, 28, 32, 33, 62
Hereford 58
Hertfordshire 28

Huntingdonshire 23
Kent 22, 29, 64
Lancashire 29, 57
Liverpool 57
London and Middlesex 20, 22, 23, 29, 32
Carpenters Hall 14
Chelsea 17
Cranford 53
Westminster 34
Monmoushire 29, 57
Llanfihangel Ystern Llewern 26
Norfolk: Norwich 58
Oxfordshire 23, 26, 33, 34
Banbury 34
Eynsham 34
Oxford 34, 54
   Bodleian Library 9
Swinbrook 34
Widford 34
Shropshire 33
Bitterley Court 31
Walcot 31
Somerset 7, 11, 13, 16, 24, 28, 29, 43, 44, 48, 51, 57, 58, 62, 63, 74
Ashton Court 29
Backwell 51
Bath 19, 57, 74
Burnham on Sea 16
Cheddar 24
Corston 26
Frome 20
Kelston 26
Keynsham, Welford House 29
Somerset, East 48
Somerset, North 33
Staffordshire 57, 70
Suffolk 23
Surrey: Dorking, Bury Hill 20
Sussex 30
Brighton, St. Nicholas 34
Lewes 34
Warwickshire 27, 29, 33, 70
Birmingham 31
Coventry 58
Foxcott 22
Westmorland 71
Wiltshire 7, 11, 13, 27, 28, 30, 48, 56, 57, 62-64, 74

Place Name Index

Wiltshire *continued*
  Corsham 64
  Malmesbury 57
  Tytherton 34
Worcester Diocese 43, 59
Worcestershire 14, 28, 31-34, 57
  Bedwardine 34
  Halesowen 62
  Wichenford 31
  Wolverley 71
  Worcester 34, 45, 58
Yorkshire 56

Wales 48, 57, 75
  Cardiganshire: Cardigan 28
  Glamorgan 29
  Radnorshire 57

Scotland 20
  Roxburghshire 27

Ireland
  Co. Wexford, Castle Annesley 23
  Dublin 23

Guernsey 24

Overseas
  Africa 15
  Australia 75
    New South Wales 16, 75
  Barbados 48
  Crimea 17
  Egypt 17
  France: Normandy 24
  Jamaica 48
  Pacific 16
  Palestine 17
  South Africa 17, 75
  United States 15, 27, 75
    Gloucester 29
  United States, Western 16

AUTHOR INDEX

ABHBA. 44, 48-52, 73
Adler, M. 63
Allen, W.T. 22, 47
Altschul, M. 23
Amey, G. 75
Anstis, R. 31
Antiquarius. 33, 61
Armitage, E.L. 36
Arundell, E. 20
Ashbee, C.R. 74
Atchley, E.G.C.F. 60, 72
Atkyns, R., Sir 8
Austin, A. 71
Austin, B. 16
Austin, R. 9, 11, 12, 17, 20, 21, 44, 45, 48, 56, 58
B., J. 35
Baddeley, W.St.C. 13, 22, 24, 40, 61, 66, 67, 69
Bagnall-Oakley, M.E. 48, 53
Bailey, W. 57
Baker, C.L.L. 38
Baker, J. 35, 56
Balch, B. 23
Bannerman, W.B. 18
Bantock, A. 29
Barclay, C.W. 20
Barclay, H.F. 20
Barker, W.R. 49
Barkly, H., Sir 20, 21, 54, 70
Barnard, E.A.B. 24, 66
Barnes, A.F. 17
Barnes, A.H. 20
Barrett, W. 8
Barron, O. 21
Bartleet, S.E. 36, 66
Bartlett, C.O. 39
Bartlett, F. 42
Barton, R. 63
Baseley, W. 68
Baskerville, G. 47, 59
Bates, C. 56
Bathurst, A.B. 20
Bayliss, W.J. 28
Bazeley, Canon 50
Bazeley, W. 9, 25, 30, 39
Beachcroft, G. 69
Beachcroft, S.P. 75

Beaven, A.B. 72
Begbie, O.M. 38
Bell, A. 74
Bellows, J. 22
Beltz, G.F. 22
Benison, W.B. 40, 42
Bergin, M. 27
Berkeley, J.H.C. 40
Bettey, J.H. 29
Bickerton Hudson, C.H. 61
Bickley, F.B. 65, 72
Biddle, D. 31
Bigland, R. 8, 50
Birch, W.D.G. 65
Biscoe, F. 42
Bishop, G.L. 44
Black, W.H. 38
Blacker, B.H. 16, 49-53
Blake, E.H. 36, 42
Blood, J.N. 38
Bloom, J.H. 35-43
Boddington, R.S. 30
Bosworth, G.F. 28
Boucher, C.E. 53
Bouth, R.H.M. 37
Bowen, E. 20
Bower, H. 21
Bradeney, J.A. 26
Bradley, A. 11
Bradshaw, T. 57
Braikenridge, G.W. 65
Bravender, T.B. 18
Bristol and Avon Family History Society 13
Bristol Public Libraries 12
Bristol Record Office. 10, 48, 72
Bristoliensis. 54
Britton, J. 61
Broad, I.R. 15
Brodigan, F. 17
Bromehead, J.N. 35, 40
Bromehill, J.N. 36
Brooke, C.N.L. 59
Brooke, G.E. 21
Brown, J. 17
Browne, A.L. 21, 31, 60, 67, 70
Bruce, J. 73
Bryans, E.L. 39, 40

Bubb, G.W. 22
Buckley, F. 15
Buckley, G.B. 15
Buckton, J.D. 61
Bullock, H. 17
Bund, J.W.W. 59
Burgess, C. 44
Bush, G. 72
Bush, T.S. 32, 66
Butcher, E.E. 72
Butler, R.F. 60
Buttrey, P. 23-25
C., R.H. 45, 53
Caine, J.M. 61
Camden, W. 18
Campbell, M.V. 37, 50
Carbonell, Canon 37
Carew, T. 17
Carlyon-Britton, P.W.P. 35
Carus-wilson, E.M. 72
Chadd, M. 23
Chapman, M.C. 33
Cheltoniensis. 49
Chitty, H. 18
Chubb, T. 18, 58
Clay, C.T. 30
Clay, C., Sir 21
Cleverdon, S. 67
Clifford, H. 23
Clifford, R. 59
Close, J. 11
Clutterbuck, J. 75
Clutterbuck, R.H. 15, 62
Codrington, R.H. 23
Coldham, P.W. 75
Commeline, Miss. 42
Conder, E. 18, 19, 67
Cooke, J.H. 21, 30, 48, 68
Cooke, R. 63
Cooper, K. 50, 53
Cordwell, J.E. 52
Corse, S.E. 61
Coss, P.R. 27
Cotterell, H.H. 16
Crawley-Boevey, A.W. 20, 69
Cripps, C. 41
Cripps, W.J. 17
Crisp, F.A. 35, 39

84

Author Index

Crisp, H. 62
Cronne, H.A. 65
D., B.C. 34
D., C.T. 18, 49, 50, 53
D., G. 54
Darwin, B. 29
Daunt, J. 23
Davenport, J. 31
Davies, G. 25
Davies, J.S. 67
Davies, W.H.S. 29, 38
Davis, C.T. 40, 48, 51, 54
Davis, U.J. 40
De Cobham, T. 59
De Havilland, J.V.S. 23
Deane, M. 24
Dennison, S. 27
Denny, H.L.L. 26
Dethick, H. 18
Deverill, P. 15
Devine, M. 69
Dickinson, M.G. 43
Dighton, C. 24, 28, 29, 39, 51
Dixon, N. 9
Douglas, A. 71
Douglas, A.W. 38
Dowdeswell, E.R. 25, 37, 42, 68
Dowler, G. 15
Downend Local History Society 56
Driver, J.T. 70
Druit, H. 51
Dudbridge, B.J. 24
Dumas, J. 37
Dunbar-Dunbar, J.A. 22
Duncan, L.L. 43, 46
Duncan, R. 75
Eales, E.F. 39
Earwaker, J.P. 53, 55
Eastwood, J.M. 67
Eberle, E.F. 15
Edwards, E.W. 35
Ellacombe, H.T. 65
Ellis, A.S. 54, 66
Ellis, M.H. 61
Elrington, C.R. 15, 54, 60
Emlyn-Jones, S. 36
Evans, J.S. 75
Evans, J.T. 38
Evans, W.J. 37
Everett, D. 70
Everett, D.M. 71
Eward, S.M. 15
Farr, G. 16

Fenwick, T.F. 18
Ferry, V. 62
Field, C.W. 59
Finberg, H.P.R. 7, 21, 46
Finberg, J. 7
Fletcher, R.J. 60
Fletcher, S. 49
Fletcher, W.G.D. 20, 24
Foliot, G. 59
Foljambe, C.G.S. 53
Fortescue, T. 24
Fosbrooke, T.D. 8, 21
Fossett, W.S. 35
Fowler, W.G. 25
Fox, F. 17
France, R.S. 66
Franklin, P. 13
Franklyn, C.A.H. 29
Franks, A.W. 48
Freeman, A.B. 14
Frere, H.C. 35
Frith, B. 33
Fry, E.A. 33, 38, 43, 47
Fry, G.S. 44, 47
Fryer, A.C. 48
Fryer, K.H. 73
Fuller, E.A. 45, 46, 55, 72
Fust, J.H. 25, 38, 50, 61
Fynmore, R.J. 27
G., B.W. 47
G., I.E. 25
G., J. 29, 51, 52
Gairdner, J. 59
Garne, R.O. 25
Garrard, E.H. 39
Gaskell, E. 13
Gaydon, A.T. 10
Gayner, M. 25
Gell, R. 57
Genealogist. 9, 44, 48
George, E.S. 43
George, W. 23
Gethen, M.A. 43
Gethyn-Jones, J.E. 37
Gibbs, H.H. 25
Gibson, J.S.W. 55
Giffard, G. 59
Ginsborough, W. 59
Gloucestershire Family History Society 12, 13, 34
Gloucestershire Record Office 10
Gloucestriensis. 28, 70, 73
Goddard, R.W.K. 53
Gomme, A. 14

Goodbody, M. 30
Goodman, W.L. 14
Goulstone, J. 24, 65
Gray, I. 10, 18, 21, 28, 37, 46, 53, 70-73
Green, A. 35
Green, J. 11
Greenfield, B. 45
Greenfield, B.W. 23, 30, 36
Greenfield, P. 71
Greening, G.H.B. 42
Greenway, D.E. 59
Greet, M.J. 14, 44, 46, 55, 66, 73
Griffin, P.K. 75
Griffiths, E.T. 36
Groome, W.I. 10
Guise, W.V. 55
H. 42, 71
H., A.W.C. 31
H., J.M. 45, 55, 59
H., R.A.G. 68
Hadfield, A.M. 7
Hadfield, C. 7
Hadow, W.E. 50
Haines, P.M. 59
Haines, R.J. 11, 22, 23, 29, 40, 55, 56, 73
Hale, R. 35
Hale, W.M. 25
Hall, I 29
Hall, I.V. 22, 23, 25, 27
Hall, J.M. 38, 40, 44-46, 54, 55, 60, 67
Hamilton, S.G. 35, 39
Hankey, J.A. 20
Hansom, J.S. 35
Harding, J.A. 62, 63
Harding, N.D. 10, 65, 72
Hardwick, N.M. 14
Hargreaves-Mawdsley, R. 75
Hart, C.E. 74
Hart, W.H. 69
Hartshorne, A. 48
Harvey, W.M. 45
Hastling, A.H.L. 75
Hayden, R. 62
Heane, W.C. 18, 26, 44, 67
Hertford, Earl of 56
Hicks Beach, W., Mrs. 26
Hicks, F.W.P. 47, 65
Hill, M.C. 32, 66
Hilton, R.H. 7, 69
Hipwell, D. 33

Historical Manuscripts
  Commission 11
Hockaday, F.S. 11
Hollis, D. 14
Holmes, M. 35
Holt, H.F. 31
Hooper, J.G. 60
Hope, S. 36
Hornsby, F.W.D. 75
Horton-Smith, L.G.H. 26
Hough, L. 43
Howes, R. 11
Hudd, A.E. 72
Hudleston, C.R. 15, 23, 25, 28, 32, 36, 54, 565, 68
Huntley, R.W. 13
Hyett, F., Sir 29, 70
Hyett, F.A. 9, 11, 16
J., D. 47
Jack, R.I. 69
Jackson, P. 16
Jackson, R. 16
Jeayes, I.H. 60, 64
Jeffcoat, R. 29
Jenner, M. 14
Jerrard, B. 16
Johnson, J. 7
Johnson, T.C. 35
Jones, B. 59
Jones, I.F. 14
Jones, P. 44
Jones, R.D. 39, 41
Jones, W. 12
Jordan, W.K. 7
Joseph, Z. 26
Kelsey, K. 38
Kempson, G.A.E. 40
Kempthorne, P.H. 43
Kennedy-Skipton, H.S. 21
Kent, B. 12
Kent, G. 27
Kent, J. 62
Kerr, J. 61
Kerr, R.J. 27
Keyte, F.H. 42
Keyte, M. 42
Killon, M.R. 33
Kimball, E.G. 70
King, G. 18
King, W.L. 62
Kingsley, N. 10, 63
Kirby, I.M. 11
Kitcat, A.P. 41
Knapp, O.G. 49

L., J. 63
Lambert, W.F.A. 35, 42, 43
Lamoine, G. 72
Lane, G.B. 26
Langston, J.N. 22, 25, 27, 29, 61, 75
Lart, C.E. 36
Latham, R.C. 66
Latimer, J. 8, 15, 32, 66, 72
Lawrence, R.G. 27
Lawson, R. 13
Le neve, J. 59
Leigh, E.E. 36
Lemmon, C.H. 13
Leotard, A. 68
Lepper, C. 75
Lewin, R. 15, 18, 51, 63
Ley, M. 50
Lillingston, E.B.C. 62
Lindegaard, P. 15, 16, 22, 29, 33
Lindley, E.S. 11, 20, 21, 25, 69
Lingen-Watson, A. 28
Little, B. 14
Little, E.C. 27
Littleton, J. 14
Livock, D.M. 72
Lloyd, W.W. 36
Lobel, M.D. 58
Longden, H.I. 27
Lowe, R. 23
Lynch-Blosse, R.C. 41
Lyne, R.E. 28, 46
Lysons, S. 52
M., J. 65
Mace, C.A. 28
Machen, H.A. 28
Macinnes, C.M. 7
Mackie, J.H. 37
Maclagan, M. 23
Maclean, J., Sir 18, 20, 21, 25, 29-32, 46, 53, 54, 56, 61, 62, 65, 66-68, 70, 72
Macray, W.D. 11
Madge, S.J. 4-37, 0, 47
Maitland, F.W. 70
Malde, H.C. 42
Manchee, T.J. 71
Mansfield, G. 10, 40, 51
Marett, W.P. 59
Marriott, C. 36
Marsh, B. 14
Marshall, C.W. 22
Marshall, G.W. 28, 46
Masse, H.J.L.J. 61

Masters, B. 10, 60
Mathews, E.R.N. 9
Matthews, H.E. 16
Matthews, W. 57
May, T. 18
Mayo, C.H. 28, 43, 54
Mayo, R. 62
Mccall, H.B. 41
Mcgrath, P. 15, 44, 72
Mcgregor, M. 14
Medland, H. 61
Mercier, J.J. 38
Messam, W. 28
Metcalfe, W.C. 18
Michell, G.B. 17, 37
Middleton, H. 74
Miller, C. 65
Mills, S. 16
Minchinton, W.E. 15, 16
Moir, E. 70
Money, W. 27
Moore, D.T. 28
Moore, J. 33
Moore, J.S. 9, 44, 54
Moore, M. 21
Moreton, Lord. 13
Morey, A. 59
Morgan, E.T. 74
Morgan, K. 12
Moriarty, G.A. 24
Mortimer, R. 62
Morton, H.E. 15
Mosley, E.R. 38, 42
Moughton, F.T.S. 28
Mullin, D. 25
Munby, A.N.L. 29
Munn, K.M. 73
Murch, J. 62
Murphy, W.P.D. 56
Myles-Hook, C. 12
N. 22
Nash, Canon 40
Neale, J.A. 64
Neale, W.G. 72
Niblett, A. 45
Nicholls, H.G. 14
Nicholls, J.F. 69
Norman, G. 14
Nott, H.E. 15, 72
O'Flynn, G. 17
Oliver, G. 62
Oliver, V.L. 28
Ollerenshaw, P. 11
Onions, K. 20

Author Index

Orme, N. 60, 74
Overy, C. 31
Owen, B. 44
Owen, L. 49
P. 69
P., A.H. 61
P., F. 33
Paget, M. 20, 23, 25, 26, 66
Painter, A.C. 54
Parker, E.M.S. 29
Parker, G. 25
Parry, H. 48, 50
Partridge, J.B. 46
Patterson, R.B. 64
Pearce, E.H. 59
Penn, S. 13
Perkins, V.R. 39, 69
Perry, D. 23
Phelps, G.F. 8
Phillimore, Mrs. 37
Phillimore, W.P.W. 24, 26, 29, 30, 37, 38, 40, 43, 46, 47, 53, 55, 62
Phillipot, J. 18
Phillipps, T. 39
Phillips, J. 15, 71
Pigg, C.H. 74
Pilkington, F. 62
Pink, W.D. 29, 46, 50
Pippet, W.A. 37
Pither, M. 22
Pitman, S. 17
Pitt, W.P. 72
Popplewell, J. 61
Porter, S. 7
Potter, A.K. 27
Pountney, W. 38
Pountney, W.J. 16
Powell, A.C. 14, 15
Powell, C. 14
Powell, G. 73
Powell, J.J. 53
Powell, J.W.D. 16
Poynton, F.J. 26, 38
Pratt, A. 35, 38, 39, 42
Pratt, R. 35, 38, 39, 42
Price, R. 16
Pritchard, J.E. 18
Pryce, G. 14, 22
R., F.L.M. 53
Ralph, E. 7, 10, 14, 33, 55, 60, 66, 70-72
Ravenhill, T.H. 35, 60
Rawes, J. 48, 49, 51, 52

Redford, J.L. 40
Redstone, A. 64
Reed, J. 57
Rendell, B. 32
Ricart, R. 72
Rich, E.E. 72
Richards, M.E. 9
Richardson, D. 15
Richardson, E.M. 12
Riemer, P. 16
Ripley, P. 7
Roberts, G. 10
Robertson, D. 75
Robertson, J.D. 13
Robinson, W.J. 48, 63
Roe, E.A. 42
Roe, M. 16
Rollison, D. 7
Roper, I.M. 48-52, 54
Ross, C.D. 69
Rowlands, E. 29
Royce, D. 39, 60, 61, 69, 73
Rudd, M.A. 66
Rudder, S. 8
Rudge, S.E. 36, 39
Rudge, T. 8
Ruffell, J.V. 68
Rusling, J.W. 35, 42
S., A.B. 70
S., C.L. 52
S., E.C. 73
S., W. 59
Sabin, A. 36, 44, 69
St. George, H., Sir 18
Sale, J. 27
Sampson, W.A. 74
Sanders, G. 25
Sargeaunt, W.T. 29
Saul, N. 7, 33
Saunders, C.D. 28
Schomberg, A. 30
Scobell, E.C. 68
Scroggs, E.S. 65
Sharp, B. 7
Sheils, W.J. 59
Sheppard, W.A. 30
Silvester, J. 40
Sinclair, A. 21
Smith, A.H. 13
Smith, B.S. 7, 9, 10, 20, 64, 70, 72
Smith, G. 73
Smith, H.U. 40
Smith, J. 55
Smith, L.T. 71

Smith, W.E.L. 59
Smith, W.F. 52
Smith, W.J. 21
Smyth, J. 10, 11, 21
Squire, Mrs. 41
Stacey, C. 13
Stanley, J. 62
Stapleton, G. 22
Steel, D.J. 33
Stenton, D.M. 70
Stevenson, W.H. 67, 73
Stilsbury, G.B. 21
Stokes, E. 47
Stone, B.G. 33
Storr, F. 74
Storr, W.R. 41
Strange, A. 73
Stratford, J. 13
Sudeley, Lord 31
Summers, P. 18
Swale, A. 48
Swynnerton, C. 30, 68
Symonds, W. 35-42, 61
Symonds, W.S. 52
T., H.Y.J. 54
Tann, J. 29
Tate, W.E. 64
Tawney, A.J. 56
Tawney, R.H. 56
Taylor, C.S. 62
Taylor, F. 64
Taylor, J. 43
Thomas, J.A. 39
Thompson, H.L. 29
Thorp, J.D. 60, 66
Till, R. 32
Todd, F.W. 26
Tonkinson, T.S. 37
Tower, F. 38
Townsend, J. 62
Tratebas, G.N. 29
Trotman, F.H. 31
Trotter, A. 43
Trotter, A.O. 37
Tudor, J.L. 42, 52
Tunnicliff, W. 57
Twining, S.H. 30
Tyndale, A.C. 31
Vanes, J. 65
Vaughan, S. 12
Veale, E.W.W. 72
Veale, T. 38
Vernon, J.E. 40
Viator. 50, 51, 54

Author Index

W., A. 61
W., H. 32
Wade, E.F. 49
Wadley, T.P. 22, 28, 40, 44-46, 60, 61
Wagner, H. 29
Wakefeld, H. 59
Walcot, M.G. 31
Walcot, P.J. 31
Walcott, M.E.C. 62
Walker, D. 64, 67, 69
Walker, F. 7
Walker, T.W. 68
Walters, H.B. 14
Ward, R.V. 75
Wardley, P. 11
Waters, R.E.C. 23
Watson, C.E. 65, 67
Watson, E.J. 70
Watts, J. 56
Way, L.J.U. 47, 65-67, 69

Way, L.U. 29
Weare, G.E. 60
Webb, F.G. 16
Webb, T.C. 43
Welch, F.B. 66, 70
Wells, C. 70
Were, F. 8, 18, 19, 54
Wherry, A. 7
Whitaker, J. 28
Whiting, J.R.S. 7
Whittard, W.F. 7
Whittington, M. 32
Wiggin, W. 38, 73
Wilkins, H.J. 17, 42, 51, 62, 74
Wilkinson, L. 39
Willcox, W.B. 70
Williams, A. 38
Williams, J. 14
Williams, J.R. 17, 75
Williams, M.E. 55
Williams, W.R. 70

Wilmot, E.A.E. 26
Wilson, J. 44
Wilson-Fox, A. 20
Wilton, J.P. 18
Winkless, D. 30
Witchell, M.E.N. 23
Witts, E.J.B. 52
Wood, J.C.N. 32
Woodman, V.A. 10, 73
Woods, S.R. 7
Woodward, G.J. 37
Woodward, J. 19
Wrigley, E.A. 41
Wyall, I. 71
Wyall, J. 71
Wyatt, I. 75
Wyllmer. 52, 60
Yarbrough, A. 14
Yescombe, E.R. 32